A Mild Traumatic Brain Injury Playbook

For Patients, Caregivers, & Physicians

Sean Patrick Mullins, MA Education

Foreward by Maureen Miner, MD

Also, By the Author

A Case Manager's Playbook
For Post-Acute Care Nursing and Rehabilitation

To my dear friend Michael J. Richter.

This playbook is dedicated to you and the brain injured clients
that you represent.

*When all hope appeared to be lost, you shared your amazing gift
to open the curtains and let the sunshine in.*

Thank you

Step into my shoes and walk the life

I'm living and if you

Get as far as I am,

Just maybe you will see

How strong I am.

Foreword

As a physiatrist who specializes in catastrophic rehabilitation, I help to direct the lifelong path in a patient with traumatic brain injury. Mild traumatic brain injury (mTBI) is an often misunderstood but very real entity, and it takes a physician who specializes in brain injury to genuinely help someone during his or her recovery. As no insult to a brain is like another, so is the response that a person with a mTBI has. A proper diagnosis is just the start. After that, a sincere and detailed delineation of problems resulting from the brain injury followed by an organized and functionally-focused treatment plan is the best way to tackle this challenging and life-changing diagnosis. For the author Sean Mullins, the writing of his book *A Mild Traumatic Brain Injury Playbook* was both an education and a journey for him. As his mTBI physician, I have seen Sean develop and optimize his own set of strategies to make him as functional and as independent as possible. In this playbook, he has been able to identify some key problems that plague many patients with this diagnosis. In essence, Sean Mullins the student learning-by-experience has become a teacher in the same, hoping that others will be able to benefit from the practical applications that he and his team of clinicians have found helpful. I am proud of my patient and this author, Sean Mullins, in his willingness to make mistakes along the way and persevere despite his disability. In my field of medicine, a person with mild TBI is often called a "walking wounded" because on the outside someone may look fine, but on the inside and every day they struggle. I pray that this book can help others better understand that there is life after a mild traumatic brain injury, and can provide some practical tools that I use in my own clinical practice to empower someone to put together his or her own "playbook" to be the best they can be. It is with admiration for this author that I endorse his manuscript.

Maureen Miner, MD
South County Pain & Rehabilitation, Inc.
Diplomate, American Board of Physical Medicine & Rehabilitation
Diplomate, American Board of Pain Medicine
Subspecialty Board Certified, Spinal Cord Medicine
Subspecialty Board Certified, Pain Medicine
Subspecialty Board Certified, Brain Injury Medicine
Qualified Medical Examiner

Table of Contents

Appendices

Figures

Head Trauma

Head trauma consists of either an open or closed injury to the brain. An **open-head injury** is defined as when the skull is penetrated. This type creates a focal injury (explained below) that affects a specific part of the brain. Open-head injuries stem from external causes such as a gunshot wound or being struck by a blunt object. An open-head injury will make the brain swell. On the other hand, with a closed injury, where the skull is **NOT** penetrated, brain damage often results from external forces that cause the brain to move within the skull.

A **closed-head injury** can be compared to a pitcher throwing a baseball into a catcher's mitt. The ball is thrown with force and may have a spinning motion before it impacts the catcher's glove. The baseball may appear to be undamaged on the outside but has tears inside its core that are not visible to the naked eye. A closed-head injury to our brain is remarkably like that baseball hitting the catcher's glove. Upon impact, the head is subjected to a violent force that jars the soft floating brain inside the interior of the skull. Sometimes the brain will experience a phenomenon called **focal injury**, where the brain rotates and stretches, strains, or tears nerve cells at the point of impact. This differs from a **diffuse injury**, where the stretching and tearing of brain nerve fibers are widespread, leading to momentarily loss of consciousness (LOC).

One of the most glaring misconceptions about **mild traumatic brain injury (MTBI)** is the simple fact that an injury can occur without making contact. For example, with whiplash, the most common of these injuries, the head accelerates and decelerates, moving the brain in two or more directions at once and tearing and stretching nerve cells throughout the brain. Further, the most current research from John Hopkins University indicates that concussions may occur through bomb blasts even without direct contact. Air pressure waves from a bomb's explosion sends signals to the brain that cause a MTBI. In addition, several other causes can trigger a MTBI. The primary cause of MTBI is called a **contrecoup brain injury**, where the head strikes a stationary object, whereas a **coup injury** is when a moving object strikes the human skull. Listed below *(Fig. 1)* are the most common secondary causes.

Figure 1: Secondary Causes of MTBI

Anoxia: the lack of oxygen supply to the brain destroys healthy cells. It is best described as a ticking time bomb, since more brain damage occurs every five minutes.

Contusion *(bruising or bleeding)*: often caused by such localized trauma as a motor vehicle accident (MVA) or sports injury. It is important to recognize that a contusion can go undetected through such conventional testing as a CT or MRI scan.

Cerebral edema: swelling from an accumulation of fluid in the intra- and/or extracellular spaces of the brain. This is a complex process whereby damaged cells begin to swell, injured blood vessels leak, and blocked absorption forces fluid to enter the brain tissue.

Intracranial pressure (ICP): the increase of cranial water into the brain. ICP will reduce blood flow and decrease oxygen that the brain receives, adding growing pressure inside the skull.

Epidural hematoma: a break of blood vessels that may clot or leak between the skull and the outer layer of the brain's protective cover (dura-matter).

Subdural hematoma (SDH): a clot or leak between the dura-matter and arachnoid matter, the brain's second protective layer.

Subarachnoid hematoma (SAH): a clot or leak between the arachnoid layer and pia matter. An SAH can be a life-threatening condition even with surgery, depending on the location and the amount of bleeding.

Intracranial hematoma (ICH): a brain bleed that will tear apart axons and white matter. Picture it as axons, which are electric impulses, as being the brain's mail delivery service carrying signals from one part of the brain to another. When these axons, or messengers, are destroyed (sheared), damaged axons will formulate into a brain injury because neurons can no longer communicate with each other.

Hemorrhage, or bleed: when torn vessels release blood into the brain's tissue. It is like flowing water leaking through a broken pipe, and the burst is so profound that the flow cannot be stopped. The bleeding around the cells can cause brain damage.

Before actual impact with the ground, the motion causes axons to begin to stretch and blood vessels to tear, and the brain's surface is rattled as it bounces up against the skull's sharp ridges. Interestingly, most mild traumatic brain injuries (MTBIs) are diagnosed as closed head injuries that reveal no signs of a fracture, and most cannot be detected through such diagnostic testing as a CT or MRI scan.

This type of injury that is being described has been labeled as the "walking wounded." From a physical standpoint, the physician may say the patient is "fine," since they can walk and talk and have a negative CT scan. Many in the medical community overlook the signs and symptoms of a MTBI, so it is understandable that family, friends, coaches, teammates, and employers make untrue assumptions because they think that there is nothing wrong with a person. Here is a list of typical judgement statements frequently made after injury:

- It's all in your head.
- She's just a drug addict, or he's using again.
- He's going through a midlife crisis.
- They're just no good at their job.

When one is struggling to cope with an internal injury, they may very well not find much support. They experience overwhelming head pain, sporadic episodes of crying for no apparent reason (a neurological condition known as Pseudo Bulbar Affect, or PBA), irritability, angry outbursts, all contributing to a lack of social support. It is no wonder why depression begins to become quite evident.

I cannot emphasize enough that the term "mild traumatic brain injury" is far from being "mild." Logically, how can an injury to the brain be considered "mild?" The following scenario can happen to any active young person.

Jenny Chung is a 29-year-old who bicycles five days per week and works full-time as a human resources representative for Google. Jenny has an active lifestyle and was recently engaged to be married in the spring. On one winter morning, Jenny's life took a sudden turn for the worse. While riding her bicycle, her front wheel slammed into a pothole, ejecting her right over her handlebars and headfirst onto the concrete. She had a recollection of the initial impact but could not recall how long she was on the sidewalk before calling for help. Once a passerby finally helped her onto the sidewalk, Jenny started to experience dizziness, nausea, and severe head pain. The pain was intense, pounding and throbbing on both sides of her head. She decided to call her significant other to drive her to the emergency room. As her husband-to-be, Cliff, drove, her nausea increased. The E/R intake nurse assessed her and immediately took her into the examination room. The physician examined her and ordered a CT and MRI scan and gave her one 4 mg tablet of Dilaudid for severe pain.

All her diagnostics were negative. The physician recommended she take two to five days off from work and take 1–2 tablets of Percocet 5/325 every 4 to 6 hours for moderate to severe head pain. He encouraged her to try Tylenol 650 mg every 6 hours and use the Percocet if the pain worsened. Her rating on the Glasgow Coma Scale was 13 out of 15.

(An important side note is that if you can walk and talk and are oriented, many physicians will decide that patients like Jenny simply need rest and pain medication. In his workup, the physician concluded that Jenny sustained a concussion.)

After taking two days off, Jenny returned to work. Her co-workers commented on how great she looked for being in such a horrible accident. Of course, Jenny looked fantastic on the outside, because she always keeps an exceptionally clean and fashionable appearance. However, the Jenny on the inside felt miserable, as the throbbing head pain would not stop. The Percocet appeared to make the pain subside, but suddenly the sides of her head would throb once again. She could not focus on her tasks at work and began to mix up her co-workers' names, prepared notes for the wrong meetings, and completely missed deadlines for projects that had been assigned to her by a supervisor who never cared for her before injury.

Jenny, now back on her bicycle, was late several times since returning to work. Her energy level was completely depleted, and she found herself unable to sleep at night. She discovered that fluorescent lighting made her nauseous. As the days went by, Jenny experienced bouts of crying and did not know why. The episodes of crying seemingly occurred for no apparent reason. She decided to follow up with her primary care physician (PCP), who, after the examination, stated that she appeared depressed and anxious. Jenny's PCP then referred her for a psychiatric consultation and cautioned her that she needed to slow down the pace of her lifestyle or she would burn out.

The Five Cognitive Domains

The tragedy behind Jenny's injury is that it is more usual than not. According to the **CDC**, two million people sustain a head injury that results in cognitive complications. A staggering 1 out of 40 will result in a lifelong debilitating impairment. As many as 75% of all MTBIs are considered "mild" by nature. It is unknown exactly how many people sustain a MTBI that are not either receiving any medical attention or are like Jenny, who did not understand the impact of her MTBI or the consequences of *post-concussion syndrome (PCS)*.

For both medical practitioners and family members to truly know how to treat or care for MTBI, understanding the "MEALS" acronym is a great place to start. "MEALS" consists of five cognitive domains:

Memory and orientation

Executive functioning

Attention

Language and communication

Sensory and motor functioning

All of these domains are at risk of being damaged when a head injury occurs. Each domain is explored in greater detail below *(Fig. 2)*.

Figure 2: Cognitive Domains

Memory and orientation: most often affected during an MTBI. Includes new learning and relearning, recall, recognition, and rote memory. Many memory disorders have their greatest impact when attention to a task is required.

Executive functioning: time management, judgement, and planning that are controlled by the frontal lobe (front of the brain). Cortical (higher) and subcortical (lower) regions of the brain are connected to the frontal lobe, so when an injury occurs it can impair awareness, insight, judgement, cognitive flexibility, rage, apathy, attention, fine motor skills, attention, initiation, planning, and behavior.

Attention: the foundation or the director that governs all the other cognitive domains. It is defined as the amount of cognitive energy that we need to donate in order to complete a specific task. Attention is controlled by two entities:

Arousal: how aroused or stirred up we are.

Velocity: how fast we can mentally process information. Impairment with attention is the most common symptom associated with an acquired brain injury. To understand more fully, close your eyes and imagine what it would be like if you suddenly could not alternate between two tasks and have either no or very little memory of what the first task was. What if your occupation requires you to multi-task, and—just like that—you no longer can maintain the speed and accuracy to complete assignments? What if background noise such as music or co-workers' social interactions interfered with your ability to read? Could you manage the frustration and anguish?

Fortunately, for many MTBI survivors, neurocognitive therapy is a viable treatment for those who have sustained an attention deficit impairment.

Language and communication: aphasia and dysarthria are the two most usual dysfunctions:

Aphasia: the loss of the ability to understand words. It is due to damage that can be located within the receptive and expressive centers of the frontal, parietal, occipital, and temporal lobes of the cerebral cortex. An aphasic patient is challenged by the fact that they know the information but cannot express it. Language interpretation channels are disrupted, and it can feel as if one is stranded on an island, all alone, with no boat ride to return to the mainland.

Dysarthria: the loss of neuromuscular control of the face, mouth, and laryngeal muscles required for speech articulation. This type of injury can be quite frustrating for a patient and so can be one of the biggest causes of irritability and impatience towards others. Happily, with speech therapy treatment, improvement is possible. Even so, deficits may linger past the first year and beyond. As for treatment strategies, it is strongly encouraged to break up the patient's goals into numerological order (i.e., 1-2-3 format) and offer praise when they demonstrate functional gains.

Sensory and motor functioning: the senses provide the very first step in thinking (cognition) and linking us to the world around us. Senses allow us to monitor and process our surroundings. The primary sensory system that we will focus on in this book is the visual system, and we will be covering it extensively in a latter section. A motor impairment secondary to MTBI, such as the ability to ambulate, postural control, and grasping objects, requires the skills of a licensed physical and occupational therapist. Interestingly enough, in many MTBI patients who sustain damage that impairs visuospatial attention, deficits in both cognitive and motor function occur.

Application: The How-to Walk-Through

An MTBI patient is fortunate to come across a doctor who can offer guidance and coping strategies. If a physician can look outside of their own preconceived notions, they may see an exhausted patient who is unable to remember but seeking answers or a patient who does not have the ability to seek those answers. Many patients can only dream about finding a physician such as Jenny's PMR (physical medicine and rehabilitation) doctor, who recently earned her MTBI Specialty Accreditation.

Jenny's doctor outlined a treatment plan that would give her the best chances for recovery. Her physician began by restricting her alcohol use and other substances that can impair memory and cognition. Secondly, Jenny, with her fiancé's assistance, were instructed to have clocks and calendars all around the house, especially in work areas, bedrooms, and, most importantly, in the backyard. As an avid gardener, she learned the hard way that she would lose track of time, making her late for scheduled events like family gatherings. A garden clock kept her from being late or missing out entirely. As a reminder to move onto the next task, Jenny was advised to set her smart phone's alarm.

One of the most challenging aspects a physician may encounter is how to counsel the patient in handling social situations. The first step is to ask others when speaking to slow down, thus allowing her to absorb small pieces of information at a time. Physicians should keep in mind that it is always best to positively reinforce with the patient that it is okay to tell others to slow down, repeat, or rephrase, if necessary, in order to ensure that they have heard the information correctly. From a patient's perspective, it is extremely helpful to have a doctor such as Jenny's, who proposes interventions that make a difference toward recovery. For comparison, if an orthopedist offers crutches or a front-wheeled walker (FWW) to a patient to ambulate after a femur fracture, it is certainly appropriate for someone who sustains an MTBI to be encouraged to use a smart phone with activated recorders with microphones, tablets, or an old fashioned notebook with pen and paper to serve as assistive devices to remember important information.

Just as a physical therapist will provide treatment for a basketball player who is recovering from a ruptured anterior cartridge ligament (ACL) injury, the doctor or speech therapist will need to provide a treatment plan for the MTBI patient who sustains a cognitive impairment. A treatment plan involves activities such as these:

Matching games, such as solitaire or Uno, which focus on both attention and concentration deficits.

Coloring activities emphasizing shapes, colors, and hand-eye coordination.

Puzzles, knitting, and hand crafts that can improve attention, concentration, and memory over time.

Having a family member or friend read out loud and recall what they have heard. For those who can work more independently, books on tape are an excellent resource.

Categorize objects by using different colors for home and work using post-it notes, different colored pens, and folders. Using colors can help with recall, especially when trying to complete a specific task.

Memory exercises are invaluable towards making significant gains and can help produce a positive outcome. First, have a family or friend show a picture and place it aside. Secondly, instruct the patient to move onto another task. In the final step, the family member or caregiver pulls out the picture and asks the patient to be as descriptive as possible in recalling the details in the picture. This exercise not only helps the patient but educates others in fully understanding their loved one's cognitive disability.

Visualization techniques is a coping strategy that can help those who have sustained memory loss. One exercise for the patient to practice is for them to close their eyes after setting down an item and picturing in their mind where they have placed it. The next step is to have them open their eyes to reinforce visualizing what the image looks like. The final step is the patient's doing a task (e.g., cleaning the kitchen sink) and, once that chore is complete, try to find the item that was originally set down.

Auditory and sensory cues (*olfactory*) can serve as another aid for the MTBI survivor. To assist with memory, have the patient touch and smell items before they place them down. This process allows them to explore what helps with recall and what does not.

The olfactory game is fun and relaxing at the same time. It is extremely easy to learn and can be quite useful in stimulating the senses. The patient will need a water-based infuser and a selected aroma. The selected aroma bottle label should be taped to cover the label. Next, once the label is concealed, start the infuser and have the patient try to identify the scent. The object of the game is to strengthen olfactory memory, as this is the first memory we use in life.

Post-Traumatic Headaches (PTH)

Although medical practitioners should consider the **MEALS** acronym, many do not, thus delaying patient treatment. This invisible injury can leave one feeling socially isolated and lead to suicidal ideations due to a lack of emotional support from family and friends. Recall Jenny's story. Because of her physical appearance, her co-workers formed the impression that she was fine, while on the inside it was a completely different set of circumstances for her. She was so overwhelmed with her head pain she could not even come close to recognizing her other medical conditions, such as

- Light sensitivity (photophobia)
- Short-term memory loss
- Depression
- Insomnia

The physician diagnosed her with depression and anxiety because her CT and MRI scans were negative. From the physician's point of view, then, Jenny's "outside" presentation, combined with her symptoms, clearly presented a case for mental health. Consequently, the outcome was a psychiatric referral for depression and anxiety.

The failure of Jenny's primary care doctor's evaluation is quite common. A thorough pain evaluation of Jenny's cervical spine and bilateral trapezius was completely overlooked. According to the American Pain Society, headaches after an MTBI can range in both pain and intensity. Trauma to the head or a whiplash injury such as Jenny's are known as **post-traumatic headaches (PTH)**. Post-traumatic headaches are injuries to the vertebrae, ligaments, neck tendons, or jaw that can cause intense pressure to the head. Typical triggers for post-traumatic headaches are

- Excessive worry
- Stress
- Fatigue
- Poor posture
- Inadequate ventilation

Clinically, they are exceedingly difficult to treat as they can present terribly, like a tension headache. A PTH differs because pain symptoms span from mild to severe and may be dull, sharp, or throbbing. A patient may describe a PTH as pain that is "24/7," meaning that they are in pain all the time. Sleep may be affected, as well. Post-traumatic headaches can be very debilitating since they can affect the ability to interact with others, to do a job, or to engage in social and recreational activities. A PTH can be combined with tension, migraines, cluster, and analgesic headaches. *Fig. 3* explores each of these four headache types and how they can impact the MTBI patient.

Figure 3: Post-Traumatic Headaches

Tension headaches described by patients as two-sided pressure that feels like someone is tightening a rope around their head. Many times, they are triggered by excessive worry, stress, overwork, poor posture, and inadequate ventilation. They usually arise late in the day and can prevent one from falling asleep. Most MTBIs are associated with tension stemming from an injury to the vertebrae, muscles, ligaments, neck tendons, or jaw joint. In countless cases, the initial injury causes muscle spasms and inflammation (injured tissues) which will subsequently cause pain. The degree of pain will vary from episodic, occurring less than 15 months, or chronic, lasting greater than 15 days per month or for more than 3 months.

Migraine headaches: aching, pulsating, throbbing sensation located between the forehead or temple that lasts from 4 to 72 hours. This pain may affect one side of the head or skull. Migraine headaches may be accompanied by nausea, vomiting, numbness, muscle weakness, photophobia (sensitivity to light), phonophobia (sensitivity to sound), or osmophilia (sensitivity to smell). Irregular meal patterns, sleep cycles, physical activity, and certain types of foods can trigger migraine headaches. Some are preceded by an aura consisting of blurred vision, flashing, or brightness. An aura can cause word-finding difficulty and impair speech or reasoning. It is important for a patient to recognize fatigue, change in mood, and excessive thirst or food cravings, as all could be a signal for an impending migraine. Sleep is usually the best medicine for those who suffer from a migraine headache. Listed below are foods that trigger or can worsen a migraine headache.

Food triggers:

Alcohol	Cured meat (such as bacon)	Pizza
Beans (except green)	Figs (especially canned)	Sour Cream
Avocados	Marinated foods	Sugar
Bananas	Nuts	Yeast-raised breads and cakes
Cheeses	Onions	Yogurt
Chocolate	Peas	

Analgesic rebound headaches: due to a withdrawal from extended usage of pain medications (**analgesic**). Think about someone who rides a stationary bike to lose weight but decides to eat chocolate cake afterwards, defeating the entire purpose. Many patients describe an analgesic rebound headache as a pain that is generalized and all over the head. Symptoms include:

- Difficulty concentrating
- Nausea
- Irritability
- Restlessness

Cluster headaches: often associated with migraine headaches. The pain can be quite intense, penetrating behind the eye, and usually affects one side of the face tracing all the way down to the back of the neck. Often the root cause is nerve damage to the neck (cervical spine). The headaches can last from 15 minutes to 3 hours, and the pain can travel from one side of the face to the other. Nicotine, alcohol, and extreme emotion can cause symptoms to reoccur.

Assessment & Treatment Recommendations

Head pain can be overwhelming for patients during the initial treatment period. A possible first step is for a trial of over-the-counter **(OTC)** medication. The biggest challenge is to avoid the high risk of rebound headaches. How can this be done? By using two different types of OTC medications. To illustrate, an intervention that provided marginal relief to our patient Jenny was a combination of an analgesic and a non-steroid anti-inflammatory **(NSAID)** medication. Her new physician, a PMR **(physical medicine and rehabilitation)** and MTBI specialist, provided her with a trπeatment of both acetaminophen **(analgesic)** and ibuprofen **(NSAID)** that initially decreased the frequency of severe head pain that Jenny was having throughout the day.

Still, severe or persistent pain may call for prescription strength medication. Physicians might use an "off the counter" approach. They may use any of the many cardiovascular medications, particularly beta-blockers and calcium channel blockers. Those reduce pain by preventing blood vessels in the head from becoming constricted, as they interfere with the transmission of nerve impulses in the circulatory and respiratory systems. Or they may use anticonvulsants and anti-depressants to reduce inflammation, relax muscles, and disrupt nerve activity and so relieve the patient's pain.

Although maintaining patience is a struggle for many before injury, it can be impossible for most people once they are injured because "trial and error treatment" from the doctor is exactly how the head pain will be treated. For this reason, a pain management assessment log will be critical not only for the patient but also for the physician if a thorough evaluation is to be achieved. **Appendix A** contains a *Pain Management Assessment Tool* for the patient to complete in order to help the physician with a thorough evaluation.

Appendix A
Pain Management Assessment Tool

Name:_____

Date:_____

Pain Site:_____

Circle the words that describe your pain:

Aching	Sharp	Penetrating
Throbbing	Tender	Nagging
Shooting	Burning	Miserable
Stabbing	Exhausting	Unbearable
Gnawing	Tiring	

Check one: Occasional ◌   Continuous ◌

What time of day is worst?
Morning ◌   Afternoon ◌   Evening ◌

Rate your pain by circling the number that describes your pain right now:

|___|___|___|___|___|___|___|___|___|___|
No   1   2   3   4   5   6   7   8   9   10+
Pain

What makes your pain better? _____

What makes your pain worse? _____

What treatments or medicines are your receiving for pain? Circle the number to describe the amount of relief the medication or treatment provides you:

Treatment (include dose): _____

No   1   2   3   4   5   6   7   8   9   10   Complete
Relief   Relief

Treatment (include dose): _____

No   1   2   3   4   5   6   7   8   9   10   Complete
Relief   Relief

Treatment (include dose): _____

No   1   2   3   4   5   6   7   8   9   10   Complete
Relief   Relief

Treatment (include dose): _____

No   1   2   3   4   5   6   7   8   9   10   Complete
Relief   Relief

Treatment (include dose): _____

No   1   2   3   4   5   6   7   8   9   10   Complete
Relief   Relief

Circle the side effects or symptoms you are having?

Nausea   Itching

Vomiting   Nightmares

Constipation   Sweating

Lack of Appetite   Difficulty Thinking

Tiredness   Insomnia

Check one: Occasional ○   Continuous ○

What time of day is worst?
Morning ○   Afternoon ○   Evening ○   Nighttime ○

Additional Notes:

_____

_____

_____

_____

_____

_____

_____

_____

Non-Drug Interventions

Non-drug interventions can be introduced to aid in alleviating head, neck, and shoulder pain. Below are explanations of a number of strategies that can be utilized rather than increasing medication or adding any form of opioid, both of which may impair cognition and slow down the recovery process.

Behavioral medicine, such as biofeedback, hypnosis, cognitive behavior therapy (CBT), and relaxation training, has proven benefits for those who suffer from chronic headaches. Regrettably, one of the biggest obstacles for psychotherapy is patient cost, as many insurance plans decline to either authorize or cover mental health services. The second stumbling block is that the patient must have the cognitive ability to follow instructions if behavior medicine is to have a positive outcome, and not all patients do have that ability.

Hypnosis can teach visualization techniques. Patients have described the experience as if their pain was a bright light that was suddenly dimmed into darkness. It can help the MTBI patient overcome the fact that the injury may have impacted their brain in a way that impairs their concentration and makes it hard for them to focus on monitoring body movement, abilities which are vital for learning the very basics.

Cognitive behavior therapy (CBT) can be significant for those who suffer from chronic head pain. CBT allows the client to experience a non-threatening environment in which they can explore the connection between cognitive thoughts, beliefs, feelings, behavior, and pain.

Relaxation techniques allow the client to reduce stress, release tensed muscles, and combat hormonal changes that can cause headaches. Yoga, meditation, and visualization are types of relaxation techniques. If introduced in a slow-paced, easy-to-understand manner, and with step-by-step instructions, this method has proven to be effective in decreasing pain, anxiety, and depression. Instructions for a relaxation modality can be given in four easy steps:

1. Find a quiet place. Breathe through your nose.

2. Inhale air naturally, where it travels filling up the lungs slowly almost as if a child is blowing up a balloon.

3. Let the air naturally release through the nose as you keep focusing on breathing.

4. If your mind drifts away, take note and refocus on breathing the air once again in and out.

Physical therapy has succeeded in reducing chronic facial, head, and neck pain. The therapist can educate the patient and caregiver on a hands-on exercise program to be done in their own home environment. Treatment may be expanded to include massage, ultrasound, or water therapy.

Chiropractic treatment is helpful in reducing MTBI-related headaches. The goal of a chiropractor is to lessen the level of pain in the affected area by manipulating the cervical, thoracic, and lumbar spine. The patient needs to fully relax the muscles in order to decrease irritation to the neck muscles, nerves, and tissues; therefore, establishing rapport with the chiropractor is important in reducing post-traumatic headaches. Rapport helps with treatment because optimum results depend on the patient's completely relaxing their joints, muscles, or pain site. If the patient does not fully relax, it is difficult for a treating chiropractor to move, twist, and realign the joints, meaning that the treatment may be less successful.

Acupuncture is strongly encouraged for those who suffer from MTBI headaches. Acupuncturists treat using either an eastern or western modality of Chinese medicine. The *Eastern, or traditional,* approach involves treating the mind, body, and soul in order to increase blood flow or circulation to the affected area. A Chinese medicine physician may say that he treats a patient by following the "Meridian." The Meridian Network is described as a pathway of circulation that channels life's energy, which is known as "qi." This pathway is what allows for energy levels (qi) to improve and chronic pain to decrease. A *Western-educated* acupuncturist practices by treating one of the over 400 pressure points. The western method is short-acting when it comes to treating head pain. In contrast, an eastern Traditional Chinese Doctor of Medicine (TCM) not only treats chronic pain but also reduces symptoms of depression, anxiety, and fatigue. A patient may not see results immediately—typically, it will take at least 24 hours to notice any signs of improvement. Most patients can anticipate treatment every 2 to 4 weeks to maintain lower pain levels and promote energy recovery. The needles are thin and are **NOT** painful. Most treatments last approximately 45 to 60 minutes, with the needles staying in the affected area for approximately 20 minutes. Soft music will be playing in the background to promote relaxation. Acupuncture is not only effective with chronic pain but can also assist with cognitive and mental fatigue, concentration, and insomnia.

Trigger point therapy is applying tender pressure to specific muscle tissues that are tight in order to relieve pain and dysfunction to other parts of the body. It specifically targets the source of pain through cycles of pressure and releases that involve self-massage. Basic guidelines for self-massage begin with the importance of saving your hands. One way is to purchase a Thera Cane or lacrosse balls. If lacrosse balls are used, they need to be placed in a long sock before applying them to the affected area. Next, expectations should **NOT** be set too high but at a pain level of 5 on a **numeric rating scale (NRS)** of 1 to 10. Massage should always be done slowly, with short repeated strokes, and the trigger point worked three to six times per day.

Note: many chronic MTBI patients experience pain in the back of the neck area. It is important **NOT** to use a penetrating tool such as a Thera Cane, as this method has the potential to rupture a vertebral artery. A better, safer technique is to let your hands be the guide. Place one hand on the back of your neck with your fingers curled on the opposite side of your posterior neck. The second hand should cup (go over) the hand stroking towards the spine. After this process is complete, switch hands to work the other side. Of course, before you begin any sort of trigger point therapy or any other type of treatment, you should always consult the attending physician, neuro psychologist, or physical therapist, then proceed, following their advice.

Appendix B, contains a set of guidelines using the Ball Massage Therapy. The healthcare professional can give a copy of these instructions to the patient.

Appendix B
Trigger Point Therapy Exercise Guidelines for the Post-Concussion Syndrome (PCS) Patient

Name: _____

Date: _____

Pain Site: _____

Trigger Point Location: _____

Ball Massage Exercise
Remember to be gentle and not overly aggressive during therapeutic exercise.

- Do ball massage 30–45 seconds at a time, 5–7 times a day (at least first thing in the morning and in the evening before bed).

- Always do ball massage before stretching.

- Expect to have soreness of the muscle during ball massage. You can add a sock over the ball to soften the ball if you have significant soreness. You may want to begin by using a tennis ball and then, if you can tolerate that, advance to a harder ball, such as a lacrosse ball.

- Drink water afterwards to flush out the "exhausts" built up in the muscles.

- Apply moist heat over the affected muscle. (You can make your own heating pad. Place 4 cups of uncooked rice in a long sock, tie it, sprinkle with a few drops of water, microwave 45–50 seconds).

Order:

1. Ball Massage

2. Moist Heat

3. Stretch

Application: The How-to Walk-Through

An MTBI survivor who suffers from post-traumatic headaches must be cognizant of environmental factors that bring about symptom-flareups. To alleviate flareups, it is advisable to find a quiet location, wear loose clothing, and practice simple visualization. Deep breathing exercises are a further help. In addition, *The ACT Coach* app, found on many smart phones, offers resources to learn mindfulness coping strategies. The ACT (Acceptance and Commitment Therapy) Coach provides written and audio tour guides through each exercise. A useful feature with this app is its breakout for obtaining goals and step-by-step instructions with dates and times, along with task-completion check-off boxes that give encouragement. The breakdown of tasks helps by teaching one how to slow down their pace, which will then increase activity endurance and decrease head pain.

Below, physicians, patients, and caregivers will find other preventative measures that will assist with decreasing post-traumatic headaches *(Fig. 4)*.

Figure 4: Preventative Measures

Documentation of each episode teaches you how to modify your environment. It is important to note the time of day, recent food types eaten, emotions, and activity level. Based on what you have documented, adapt to your environment. You can change your diet by eliminating foods that seem to trigger headaches (a diet low in sugar and carbohydrates and high in green vegetables and protein is strongly encouraged) or change the pace of your activity.

Keeping a scheduled routine that consist of a regular sleeping pattern, exercise, and meal schedule. In fact, an exercise consisting of aerobic activity is excellent for releasing the brain's endorphins. **Endorphins** are the body's chemicals that interact with the brain's receptor that reduces the perception of pain.

Barometric pressure can have an impact on one's physical condition. It is important for professionals, patients, and caregivers to recognize that wet and cold weather can exacerbate headaches. If you are considering travel, choose to visit places located at sea-level, since being in high altitudes increases the frequency of headaches.

Fluorescent lighting and flashing lights are stressors that may cause eye strain, a known trigger for post-traumatic headaches. Avoiding fluorescent lighting or flashing lights is beneficial. If you experience eye strain, you should be referred to neuro-ophthalmology for further evaluation.

To be very clear, MTBI patients **must** be aware of their environmental surroundings. At the first sign of head pain or a migraine headache, changing to a much calmer and more relaxed environment is in order. It is essential to be aware of what messages (signals) the body is trying to send. Once head pain is triggered, lying down and trying to go to sleep is the first measure to take. Sleep is often the best medicine, especially in an environment away from noise.

Recalling our patient Jenny, she is now finally receiving treatment from physicians who are aware of her condition. Her PMR doctor, who specializes in treating MTBI, has counseled her to set boundaries. Her fiancé helps her, in particular by keeping her from being in an enclosed, noisy place, which makes her head feel like someone is smashing it like a hammer on concrete. Jenny's fiancé still struggles with her condition but is coming to understand that her pain is not visible and that there is much more involved in working toward her recovery.

Motor Function Problems & Poor Balance

Coordination of movement is managed by multiple areas in the brain. As compared with a stroke, where the damage is more localized, brain trauma finds its roots spread out through various sections of the brain. Depending upon the impact, the patient may have slow, jerky uncontrolled movements. Or they may experience tremors that cause such challenges as signing their name, walking up a flight of stairs, or cutting a rose stem with a pair of clippers. Again, remember Jenny. She told her doctor that, while playing the piano, midway through a song her hands began to tremor. Her complaint that the brain and the hands failed to work in unison with each other is quite common. As a matter of fact, the symptoms she was exhibiting may be a result of damage to either the parietal lobe, cerebellum, or brain stem.

Many MTBI patients are affected by muscle tone (the tightness of when a muscle is at rest). The impact of tight muscles often indicates a central nervous system (CNS) motor impairment that can cause the following symptoms to occur:

> **Muscle spasms:** the tightening of a single muscle or muscle group.

> **Hypertonicity:** tensing of all muscles, causing limbs and the trunk to stiffen.

Many healthcare providers have difficulty determining a diagnosis, as it is exceedingly difficult to establish if the muscle tone is associated with a muscle injury or brain injury.

Dizziness, vertigo, and disequilibrium are medical conditions that are quite common but frequently overlooked by physicians. Definitions of the conditions will provide a framework for an accurate diagnosis.

> **Dizziness:** a sensation of light-headedness, faintness, or unsteadiness when standing.

> **Vertigo:** the perception of rotational movement or whirling of the self or surrounding objects. Surroundings seem to spin and nausea may occur.

> **Disequilibrium:** a feeling of being off-balance or a sensation of spatial disorientation.

A balance disorder signals that the accident may have caused damage to the inner ear, which causes dizziness, vertigo, or disequilibrium. This is called a **peripheral vestibular disorder.** Patients noticing these problems must be their own advocate and request a referral to a neuro-otolaryngologist for an evaluation, although vestibular testing may be conducted by an audiologist or physical therapist, too.

As a patient, you can help your doctor make a diagnosis and determine a treatment plan by providing specific information. Think about what you are experiencing. Either jot down your responses or have a family member assist you in writing them down. Be as detailed as possible. The more your doctor knows about what you are going through, the more effective treatment plan will result. Describe your dizziness or balance problems in these terms:

- How often do you feel dizzy or have trouble keeping your balance?

- Have you ever fallen? If so, when, where, how often, and under what circumstances?

- List all of the medications you take.

Application: The How-to Walk-Through

Regrettably, most MTBI survivors do not seek treatment for muscular or motor problems unless they are evaluated by a physician's "naked eye." The naked eye for our purposes is defined as what happens to be physically visible, such as broken bones, bruises, and cuts. The problem is that MTBI usually is not thoroughly evaluated until many months after the injury. Typically, muscle tone and balance problems are worked up by a referring doctor who is either a neurologist or a PMR (pain management and rehabilitation) physician who specializes in MTBI or chronic pain.

Physical therapy can help with overcoming motor difficulties and chronic pain. A physical therapist (**PT**) can treat:

- Balance
- Motor coordination
- Muscle movement
- Spasm
- Tone
- Strength

Moreover, physical therapy uses tools that are very effective with inflammation and myofascial pain. For example, a physical therapist can utilize deep tissue modalities such as massage and e-stim therapy. An e-stim device is a small machine that has two plug-in channels attached to a cord and pads that are applied to the affected site. To a patient, e-stim feels like a very quick tap. It will be used for about 15 to 20 minutes during the treatment session. Outside the therapist's office, the patient can anticipate a home exercise program that will include range of motion (**ROM**) stretches to the head, neck, and shoulders. For use at home, TENS (transcutaneous electrical nerve stimulation) Units, H-Wave, or other e-stim devices may be added to the treatment. Although these units are made available online through such sites as Amazon.com, and it is always best to be proactive with your care, do **NOT** attempt to utilize an e-stim unit without the proper instructions from either your treating doctor or physical therapist. The healthcare professional will be able to give specific instructions on pad placement and treatment duration. It is important to recognize that the goal here is to provide neuro re-education to the affected site by decreasing inflammation and increasing muscle function, so it is critical to use these devices properly.

Chiropractor adjustments are another method that does not involve the use of NSAIDs (non-steroid anti-inflammatory drugs). They increase blood flow and nerve-impulse supply to the problematic muscle. This approach allows for freer movement of the neck, head, and shoulders while providing more space within the joints. As discussed previously, the patient must be able to trust the treating chiropractor for a successful myofascial release or the treatment will not be as effective. And they must practice being patient, because there may **NOT** be an immediate sense of relief right after the adjustment. This is due to the fact that relief created by the release of blood flow to the problematic muscles may take 2–3 days after the treatment day. Using mindfulness practices is strongly recommended if anxiety increases over the effectiveness of chiropractic care.

Here are some other helpful tips:

1. Do **NOT** jump right out of bed in the morning, but roll out slowly.

2. Try sleeping without a pillow so that your neck and upper spine remain perfectly straight and are not pushed forward.

3. Limit your use of salt, which tends to cause fluid retention and increases vertigo.

4. Avoid nicotine products such as cigarettes and vaping, along with recreational drugs, since many of these substances promote dizziness.

5. Sit or stand up slowly so you do not set off the receptors in the inner ear that will make your condition worse.

6. Be aware of medications that you are taking, as some may make you more sensitive to side effects like dizziness.

7. Notice your environmental surroundings, such as bright lights, sunlight, and noise, which can all be triggers for dizziness. Take steps to limit or avoid these conditions.

8. Most importantly, when you notice the first signs of dizziness, either sit or lie down, as this has a good chance of calming your symptoms.

Hearing Problems

In some instances, brain trauma is centered around the temporal and parietal lobes that are linked to ear function. When damage occurs to these regions of the brain, ear-related functions like balance and spatial awareness or the interpretation of sound may become impaired. However, many of the hearing problems associated with an MTBI are the consequence of damage to the middle or inner ear. Sometimes the ear drum ruptures or there is swelling to the eustachian tube (a drainage tube that connects the ear to the throat), causing the middle ear to bleed. As a result, a sound-blocking fluid begins to build up that can impact what one can hear. Similarly, tiny sensitive bones on the middle ear may hinder sound transmissions. If the cochlea or the surrounding nerve muscles bear the point of impact, hearing loss may become a permanent disability. Even worse, one may become unable to interpret auditory messages.

A hearing loss is nerve damage or a malfunction in the conduction of sound waves to the ear. When an MTBI patient encounters hearing loss, low-volume or high-pitched tones become hard to hear and rapid or monotone dialog may become difficult to understand. Hearing loss can make one feel frustrated and socially isolated, especially when placed in social situations. Fortunately, although hearing loss may become permanent, most types are treatable.

Trauma to the head and neck can result in interfering with variety of the most common perceived perceptions of external sound. This medical condition is called **tinnitus**. Patients will complain of such symptoms as ringing and buzzing noises, roaring and hissing, or high-pitched tones. Tinnitus is a problem that can worsen at night or in a quiet environment. It can be quite stressful and a nuisance. On a positive note, though, tinnitus may resolve over time.

If tinnitus had a "big sister" it would most definitely be **noise sensitivity**. A sound selection problem can occur in which one loses the ability to distinguish between certain sounds or filter out background noise. Such as in the case of our patient Jenny.

Jenny was completely lost when following dialogue in her work meetings after her injury. Her PMR physician discovered that one of her conditions was noise sensitivity. Further compounding her problems was tinnitus, a sound-selecting problem that is triggered by noise sensitivity. Jenny often felt tired and frustrated because she could not hear while driving in a car or trying to watch her favorite TV show on Netflix. Her fiancé did not understand, and his sarcastic remarks did not help the situation. . . "Why can't you hear?" "You fell on your head, maybe it's your sinuses?" "I'm tired of repeating myself." His actions are understandable. After all, if Jenny was struggling to cope with her symptoms, imagine the difficulties her significant other may be having at this point in her recovery.

Another, rare MTBI-related hearing disability is being incapable of comprehending everyday sound, a condition known as sound agnosia. **Sound agnosia** is brain damage located in the temporal parietal area of the brain's right hemisphere that leaves one able to participate in a conversation, but unable to identify background sounds such as a ringing doorbell, a dog's bark, or a crying baby. Sound agnosia can pose a significant obstacle to everyday functioning and can result in total hearing loss.

Application: The How-to Walk-Through

Many hearing disorders can be lifelong. One of the hardest-to-live-with aspects of post-injury is the brain's failure to filter out irrelevant or unnecessary information. Take a moment and imagine what life would be like if you could not filter out sounds, smells, or feelings. Imagine entering an enclosed space, maybe a grocery store or restaurant, and your sensitivity to background music or fluorescent light causes your brain to shut down. Your auditory system becomes so overwhelmed with sound that you can no longer tolerate it. The social interaction is either moving too fast for you to follow, or ear ringing and posterior head pain are so bad that you just want to leave. Before you know it, fatigue kicks in full-force, and the brain just wants to shut down. These signs and symptoms, known as **hyperacusis**, may cause you to leave your house only when places are not crowded or noisy.

One accommodation is the use of special custom-made noise dampening ear filters (**ER 15/25**). These earplugs are typically for musicians to drown out background music in order for a soloist to hear their vocals, but in the MTBI world they have been quite a useful intervention for those who have hyperacusis. The sole purpose of these ear filters is to drown out background noise, allowing a person to engage in the tumultuous world.

If hearing loss occurs from damage to the ear drum or inner ear surgery, medication can be ordered by the physician. Antibiotics and decongestants have been known to assist with reducing middle ear build-up and improve hearing loss.

Tinnitus is extremely challenging to treat, since it can be accompanied by hearing loss. Actually, a healthcare provider may find that treating hearing loss can make the tinnitus worse. But an antidepressant can be used to decrease stress or anxiety. It is important to assess all medications the patient is taking and make it clear that those taken with alcohol will make the tinnitus flare up. Proper medication adjustments may effectively decrease the ear buzzing and ringing sounds. Another intervention, highlighted above, are tinnitus-masking devices such as ear filters or hearing aids. These masking devices can minimize the long-term effects of hearing loss by reducing background noise so the patient can make a valid attempt to socially interact with others. **EEG biofeedback** is another tool that can help by consciously altering brain waves that perceive sound.

Other extremely valuable interventions are available to the patient who is challenged by ear-ringing. **Psychotherapy** provides the emotional support and interventions patients need to cope with the signs and symptoms of tinnitus. **Mindfulness-based** practices have proven to be beneficial to help the patient to relax. **Acupuncture** can be helpful in increasing blood flow and decreasing stress in order to lessen symptoms. Patients are strongly encouraged to search for a licensed acupuncturist who is certified in their state and specializes in Traditional Chinese Medicine (TCM).

As is often the case with MTBI symptoms, time is important when defining the longevity of hearing problems. While your doctor may have several recommendations for treatment, there are a few steps you can take to minimize hearing problems:

1. Avoid nicotine, caffeine, alcohol, and recreational street drugs, as they will intensify your symptoms.

2. Limit your use of salt, which can cause fluid retention and increase vertigo. Make sure to read labels at the grocery store when you shop and check for foods low in sodium.

3. Keep a regular sleep schedule to reduce stress and anxiety.

4. Sleep with a radio playing, an electric fan, or a baby monitor to minimize the effects of tinnitus. Plenty of apps are available for smart phones. A useful one, *Relax Melodies* by Ipnos, offers a variety of soothing sounds designed specifically for this purpose.

5. Call your local phone company's customer service to inquire about special audio equipment that can make conversing through text easier by displaying the words on an LCD screen.

6. Do **NOT** be shy with regards to your hearing loss. It is okay to say, "Excuse me. Can you please speak one at a time?" or "Can we find a quieter place to talk?"

7. Take care of yourself by avoiding large group functions, especially those that are enclosed and have an echo effect. If possible, shop during off-peak hours, such as between 8:00 am and noon. Select a store that does not have music playing at high volumes. Be open to asking family and friends to help, especially during the earlier phases of recovery.

8. If you find yourself extremely anxious or depressed regarding your hearing problems, ask the physician for resources for support or professional psychological help.

Vision Problems

Even though it is quite obvious when there is head and neck pain or memory problems, we may not associate vision problems with them. Yet, many MTBI survivors do have difficulties with their eyes. The most commonplace complaints are double and blurred vision. There is, though, a wide range of modalities, from partial vision loss, to tracking (**difficulties focusing on moving objects**), to photophobia (**sensitivity to light**). After the brain sustains damage from the force and impact of hitting a surface, it will be very difficult for the doctor to predict whether or not normal vision will be restored.

Vision is a complex, delicate process. The eyeball and optic nerve are vulnerable to a variety of injuries. Sometimes the eyeball itself sustains an injury that can bend, compress, twist, and jolt the retina and/or optic nerve. In other cases, the skull or the back of the neck may damage delicate tissues in the brain stem that regulate eye coordination and movement. It may just take a blow to the top of the head to cause damage to the parietal lobe and affect higher-level skills such as reading. It cannot be repeated enough to patients that they should try to pinpoint the root of any vision problem and urge their primary care physician to refer them for an evaluation by a **neuro ophthalmologist,** who specializes in the care of vision problems associated with neurological disorders such as MTBI.

Back to Jenny, who is a prime example of someone having to deal with vision problems after an injury. Over time, Jenny encountered problems with blurred vision that were worsened by stress and fatigue. On occasion, she was confronted with fluorescent lighting that caused nausea and headaches. Her problems were ones that are exceedingly difficult for a physician to treat, since corrective or prescribed lenses do not make her symptoms any better. As a result, Jenny learned to stay away from such conditions and purchased a pair of special over-the-counter glasses that helped with reducing her symptoms of nausea and headaches caused by fluorescent lighting.

Healthcare providers must not limit themselves to one diagnosis but be open to many. **Blurred vision,** or seeing objects out of focus, can be problematic. This can happen when there is damage to the cornea or to the optic nerve, which transmits visual messages to the brain. With blurred vision, everything is out of focus. Some cases of blurred vision heal over time, but in others, especially if there is retinal or optic nerve damage, one may be left with a permanent disability.

Another diagnosis, **cortical blindness,** can be described as the "evil stepsister" to blurred vision. Often caused by damage to both occipital lobes, the disability can vary from complete blindness to an inability to read small or medium size print. Frequently, the occipital lobes will heal and vision is restored, but cortical blindness may result in full vision loss.

Under normal conditions, the eyes are synchronized where both retinas can focus on a single picture. When nerve damage occurs, the retinas will see each image separately. This phenomenon is called **diplopia**, or double vision, where one distinct vision becomes two images. Double vision may worsen when symptoms such as head and neck pain, fatigue, and dizziness are triggered. Diplopia can disappear within 6 weeks from injury or may become permanent, depending upon the severity of the nerve damage.

Again, healthcare providers should not hesitate to make a referral for neuro ophthalmology, especially when seeking an evaluation to rule out **optic atrophy.** If the optic nerve can no longer transmit impulses from the retina to the brain, the patient may have blurred vision. Optic atrophy may be the cause of faulty depth and distance perception after an injury. Diagnosis and treatment of optic atrophy requires the skills of an astute neuro ophthalmologist who will examine the patient's optic nerves. This evaluation will require the patient to be calm and relaxed during the exam, so patients should be advised to practice mindfulness or prescribed a one-time dose of an anti-anxiety medication before the exam. Furthermore—and this cannot be emphasized enough—it may take time for the patient to become fully aware of their symptoms, so if there are any vision problems that the patient reports, the treating physician should seriously consider recommending a neuro-ophthalmologist sooner rather than later.

Although unusual, another medical condition resulting from injury to the visual system is **photophobia,** or sensitivity to light. Photophobia can manifest itself as an annoying glare from certain types of light, such as fluorescent. Light sensitivity can trigger headaches and nausea. Photophobia can be either a short-term problem or a chronic condition, depending upon the type and severity of the injury.

Tracking, or the ability to maintain focus on an object, can be problematic for MTBI survivors. Tracking problems may be the result of a brain stem or cerebellum injury. A brain stem injury can sometimes cause **nystagmus,** or rapid oscillations of the eyeball. Nystagmus interferes with the eye moving up and down and left to right, and it slows the eye movement, making it difficult to read and process information.

Visual overstimulation and **visual field changes** are two medical conditions that are seen in brain injured individuals. Visual stimulation is when light patterns and/or viewing movement and color interfere with the ability to process information. This condition is tied to one or more parts of the brain that endured trauma after the injury. The recovery rate is unpredictable, from short- to long-term and from mildly to completely incapacitating. Visual field changes impair a portion of either the peripheral or central and side eye-site when looking straight ahead. This is what can be called "visual field cuts." A **visual field cut** is when one can see out the center but has either blurred vision or an inability to see from left to right. Many global factors are in play here, but the root of the problem is most likely found in an injury to both occipital lobes or to the optic nerve.

Application: The How-to Walk-Through

As with other parts of the body, when the brain sustains an injury there can be improvement over time. If one's vision is blurred, an ophthalmologist may offer vision rehabilitation. Looking once again at Jenny, her experience explains how **vision rehabilitation** applies to an MTBI patient with visual field deficits. She had blurred vison in the left eye as a result of her injury. Her ophthalmologist advised her, when reading, to hold the printed matter to the right of her nose, therefore compensating by using the stronger side of her visual field. This helped Jenny be able to read without seeing blurred lines.

Physicians might order an antibiotic and/or anti-inflammatory medication such as prednisone, especially if there is damage to the cornea. The purpose is to produce **protein TSG-6**, which has been shown to reduce **corneal opacity** (scarring that reduces light, causing the cornea to become white in color) and **neovascularization** (growth of new blood vessels, depriving oxygen to the cornea and thus harming eye site). Studies have shown that, after a course of 21 days of treatment, patients show vast improvements from the point of injury (Joo Youn Oh, Gavin W. Roddy, Hosoon Choi, Ryang Hwa Lee, Joni H. Ylöstalo, Robert H. Rosa, Jr., and Darwin J. Prockop, *Anti-inflammatory Protein TSG-6 Reduces Inflammatory Damage to the Cornea Following Chemical and Mechanical Injury.* 2010. PNAS 107 (39) 16875-16880).

Many MTBI survivors suffer from light sensitivity or visual overstimulation. If so, the doctor may advise ways (**compensatory techniques**) to avoid pain and distressful visual stimulation. Special glasses with either dark or orange lenses, such as the **TheraSpecs** (www.theraspecs.com), are available over the counter or can be purchased online. Using computer tint screens and encouraging the patient to work in a room with the blinds down may eliminate unnecessary shading. A person can wear a hat in order to block out lighting that is a nuisance. Avoiding chaotic places and shopping during off-peak hours is a preventative, as is avoiding shopping malls with their drastic contrasts in lighting and noises from one store to the next. Healthcare professionals should evaluate the patient for dry eyes, as this is not only associated with brain injury but can be a side-effect of medications. The patient may need an over-the-counter or prescription eye lubricant to help alleviate the problem. And anyone who finds themselves in a fragile emotional state over their visual problems should **NOT** hesitate to ask their attending physician for a referral to counseling or mental health so that the treatment and healing process can be more effective.

Convergence insufficiency is a condition that causes one eye to turn outward instead of inward with the other eye, creating double or blurred vision. It is the cause for eye strain and headaches associated with a post-concussion syndrome (PCS). The doctor may prescribe exercises to help train the patient's eyes to hold close views for longer periods of time. One such exercise is to insert a golf tee into a straw or pegboard. Or the doctor may utilize the patient's occupation as part of treating convergence insufficiency. A carpenter would be asked to gently hammer a nail, or a nurse might be asked to practice injections into an orange. Such exercises are easy to do at home and help reduce blurred vision. They may feel tedious and frustrating at first, but they are a positive step forward.

Fatigue

Fatigue is the second most commonly identified symptom, occurring three times more often than in the non-brain injured person, and it is least treated by medical professionals. Family members may mistake fatigue as being rude during family functions, or lazy, or being overly medicated. Once again, such reactions are understandable, considering that physicians themselves overlook fatigue when considering a treatment plan for the MTBI patient.

Before an injury, a healthy brain will perform a multitude of physical, emotional, and cognitive activities and still have the reserve to function throughout the day. For example, Jenny was able to multi-task very well prior to her injury. She participated in several work-related meetings throughout the day for Google. Then, after her injury, her brain did not have the energy to support cognitive or emotional issues, leaving little or no reserve. No matter what Jenny did in the afternoons, she lacked the mental stamina to complete such simple tasks as filing case numbers. Her ability to concentrate, along with her memory and sense of motivation, was sluggish and out of step. She tried caffeine, carbohydrates, and sugary snacks, but they did not give her the second wind she needed. She felt as though she were moving one step slower than real time, and she began to feel the need to lie down. As she told her doctor, everything appeared heavy and confusing, and she was left feeling spacy and faint. What occurred with Jenny is not at all unusual for the brain injured, as the brain uses more energy than any organ in the entire body and has a pool of reserve that will keep one from overextending themselves. From a patient's perspective, it is as though the pool of reserve has gone from a lap pool to a hot tub, requiring much more energy to perform basic functions throughout the day. The energy reserve is basically non existent, and when one pushes themselves too much, extreme fatigue may cause the brain and body to shut down. In turn, this exhaustion can intensify symptoms and be the root cause for an emotional reaction. Frustration begins to mount as one cannot complete tasks. Walking, driving, and coordination of movement become severely limited and can place either the patient or others around them at risk.

Many patients struggle with concentration, reading, writing, and problem solving. Putting forth an effort causes mental and cognitive fatigue. The simplest tasks become daunting. Balancing a checkbook, driving, writing, and social interaction take great effort. Fatigue spirals into slow processing of information, such as following simple instructions, and difficulty maintaining attention. The person feels that they are in a fog. This **"brain fog"** is when your energy level is so low that everything appears to be grainy and looks like one big blur, much like a person who has perfect vision trying to wear their friend's prescription eyeglasses. In the morning, you may say that you will be able to perform various tasks, but then you notice a drop in energy around 12 noon or 1:00 p.m. in the afternoon. Or fatigue begins to set in when you are overstimulating at a social event. And a couple hours in an enclosed area such as a shopping mall with different types of lighting, noises, and crowds of people are an energy nightmare for the MTBI patient.

Mental fatigue is frequently a trigger for physical fatigue, which can start with severe head and neck pain and be followed by an overwhelming desire to sleep. The eyes become heavy and stop allowing further processing of information, and people in the MTBI world will say that they are "blown." Individuals who suffer from mental fatigue experience a profound disability that impacts not only their work function, but also their overall capacity to participate in social activities for years after the brain injury has occurred.

Application: The How-to Walk-Through

A cognitive and mental fatigue treatment plan must be patient centered and specific, because each patient's brain chemistry is impacted differently by their injury. The first factor to consider is side effects to medications, weighing the risks against the benefits regarding the patient's level of fatigue. Does the scheduled dosage cause additional fatigue, or does it treat the patient's pain so they can perform at their highest practical level? As time consuming as this determination may be during an evaluation, it is important. The patient's medication list should be discussed and reviewed, and if there is an alternative to either reduce or trial a new medication, this needs to be considered. If this does not happen, the patient, family, and caregiver can request a pharmacy consultation and bring the information to the next doctor's appointment.

Sleep patterns should be reviewed and further explored. It is important that MTBI patients get at least 6–10 hours of sleep per night. This can be achieved by not drinking any fluids past 8:00 p.m. so as to avoid having to awaken for urination. Going to bed at the same time each night will improve sleep habits. Avoid taking naps during the day, as this will wreak havoc on your sleep pattern at night. Conversely, if the fatigue is overwhelming toward the brink of exhaustion, it is fine to take one nap midday.

Coping with physical fatigue may mean prioritizing daily tasks so that the most cognitively complex responsibilities are scheduled for the morning when the mind is fresh. Avoid getting overtired, as this can set you back for days. Utilizing a pacing method can help keep you from becoming overtired. Pacing activities requires you to break an activity up into active and rest periods. Rest periods should be taken before pain increases. Research has demonstrated that it is best to utilize a window between 3:00 a.m.–12 noon and 6:00 p.m.–8:00 p.m. to perform the most brain-tasking functions. The goal is to minimize pain and maximize productivity during the day. When you feel an increase in symptoms, such as head pain and fatigue, document and share it with your provider. If your symptoms continue for greater than 2 hours and at a rate greater than a 3 out of 10 on the numeric rating scale (NRS), it is extremely important that the physician be made aware.

An effective assessment tool for the medical practitioner's evaluation of fatigue can be found in **Appendix C.** *The Fatigue Severity Scale (FSS)* is a 9 item assessment scale that measures *global fatigue*, the severity of fatigue and how it impacts a person's activity and lifestyle.

Appendix C
Fatigue Severity Scale (FSS)

Name:_____

Date:_____

Please circle the number between **1** and **7** which you feel best fits each statement. This refers to your usual way of life within the last week. **1** indicates *strongly disagree* and **7** indicates *strongly agree.*

Circle the appropriate number for each statement	Strongly Disagree ←——————→ Strongly Agree						
1. My motivation is lower when I am fatigued.	1	2	3	4	5	6	7
2. Exercise brings on my fatigue.	1	2	3	4	5	6	7
3. I am easily fatigued.	1	2	3	4	5	6	7
4. Fatigue interferes with my physical functioning.	1	2	3	4	5	6	7
5. Fatigue causes frequent problems for me.	1	2	3	4	5	6	7
6. My fatigue prevents sustained physical functioning.	1	2	3	4	5	6	7
7. Fatigue interferes with carrying out certain duties and responsibilities.	1	2	3	4	5	6	7
8. Fatigue is among my most disabling symptoms.	1	2	3	4	5	6	7
9. Fatigue interferes with my work, family, or social life.	1	2	3	4	5	6	7

Visual Analog Fatigue Scale (VAFS)
Please mark an "X" on the number which describes your global fatigue, with **0** being *worst* and **10** being *normal.*

1	2	3	4	5	6	7	8	9	10

Pacing

Pacing can bring many benefits to the patient, like structure and a sense of control. However, the biggest task for the treating provider is to slow the patient down, to keep them from rushing once they become frustrated when tasks may take two or three times as long as they anticipated. They can acknowledge their limited thinking capacity, but using it wisely is easier said than done, especially if, prior to the injury, operating in a fast paced environment was their forte. They want to function and complete tasks as they did before. In the past, they may have been able to manage many tasks at once with plenty of set-shifting but now have flareups that create fearsome hurdles.

Flareups may result from increased head pain or tinnitus A patient may feel angry and helpless and struggle with maintaining calm. The primary treating provider should incorporate a psychologist or social support system into the treatment plan to help the patient find this calm. Secondly, the provider will need to gradually educate the patient on a pace method that will maximize their cognitive ability in order to reduce fatigue. The first step is incorporating a pace method with **instrumental activities for daily living (IADLs)**. IADLs may include such household chores as mopping the kitchen floor, preparing meals, or cleaning the bathroom. A common pace method is described below:

Pace Method:

5 minutes of mopping the kitchen floor

    10 minute break

5 minutes mopping the kitchen floor

    10 minute break

5 minutes of mopping the kitchen floor

    10 minute break

5 minutes mopping the kitchen floor

Even if the activity takes longer, the goal is to decrease the number of flareups by decreasing pain and increasing activity tolerance. The MTBI patient will face dangers here, such as having a great start to the day and becoming overconfident. Overconfidence in the MTBI world can work as a disadvantage, resulting in the patient's exerting much more than they should. This will bring on flareups that can be physically, mentally, and cognitively exhausting. As another example, they may try to please family members by participating in functions that will only make their condition worse. They need to be proactive by incorporating a pace method and giving themselves permission to tell their family members what they can tolerate and why they either will have to leave early or find a quiet place to rest.

Application: The How-to Walk-Through

Patients can establish pacing by setting up blocks of time for work and breaks before flareup begins. Physicians should take note that this may cause the patient to become frustrated, so it is important that they be educated on how to remain calm. Once more, Jenny's experience can illustrate this. She began her pacing by starting one activity in the early morning, when most MTBI survivors are the freshest from a cognitive standpoint. After a number of trial runs that resulted in several flareups, she realized that her speech therapist's writing exercises could be broken up into 10 minute segments, followed by 5 minute breaks. She tried this pattern but alternated the writing exercises with household tasks and practicing her breathing exercises. Soon she saw a benefit from taking a 15 minute break from her writing tasks after she completed two sets of 10 minutes of writing and 5 minutes of household chores. She then incorporated exercise into her daily routine, with the guidance of her PMR physician. In short, Jenny developed a personalized pacing pattern that yielded significant benefits for her.

Exercise has proven beneficial not just to Jenny but to many others who have sustained a MTBI. Physical activity increases vascular blood flow, reduces depression and anxiety, improves sleep, and promotes neuroplasticity by regenerating nerve cells **(neurons)** that improve memory and thinking. Research has shown that people with MTBI who exercise have fewer cognitive complaints of irritability, forgetfulness, and being disorganized. *Note: patients who are interested in exercise, must consult with their physician prior to beginning, especially those who have problems with balance or memory that may endanger their safety.*

Additionally, physician involvement is critical for a successful outcome, as exercise should be increased only as tolerated. It is important for a treating provider to tailor an exercise program to a patient's specific overall needs and abilities. Many MTBI survivors are unable to drive or have sustained physical or cognitive limitations. The inability to drive may leave the patient with no choice but public transportation, ride sharing, or a home based exercise program. But modified selection of exercises/machines, group/club activities, and adaptive sports/recreation are all viable options. Equally important is focusing on both aerobic exercise (e.g., swimming or running) and non aerobic exercise. Yoga, Tai Chi, weight training, bowling, and golf can all promote relaxation and improve concentration. Identifying what exercise resources are available in the patient's surrounding area is key. Possibilities include Parks and Recreation, the YMCA, health clubs, independent living centers, adult education classes, and the local or state **Brain Injury Association**.

If there are memory issues, keeping index cards that contain specific steps in an activity is helpful. This requires an activity that has a structured routine that will allow handwritten step-by-step instructions. Smart phone technology is quite useful, especially with apps that provide pictures with step-by-step guides through an activity and alarms that help patients stay on task. Paper calendars can promote successful outcomes, too, especially as reminders of dates and times and when specific exercise is scheduled.

An MTBI exercise program should consist of three components. The first is *cardiovascular*, which is meant to increase heart rate and keep the muscles strong. Cardiovascular activity impacts the heart, lungs, circulation, and muscles. Walking/jogging on a treadmill, pedaling on a stationary bike, water aerobics, and dancing are examples of cardiovascular exercises that a treating provider might recommend to a patient.

Secondly, a *strengthening* program should be considered that will strengthen muscles by pushing and pulling against resistance. Bone density, balance, and posture will all see an improvement over time. Free weights, resistance training machines, and tubing/bands are examples of strengthening exercise methods. Most treating physicians or physical therapists will emphasize a routine strengthening exercise program for the head, neck, and shoulders.

Lastly, a program that promotes *relaxation* by increasing muscle length and improving range of motion can reduce tension headaches and improve range of motion. Improved flexibility will make it easier to get into positions such as squatting, bending, or reaching. As mentioned above, a treating provider may encourage patients to engage in yoga and Tai Chi, especially those who have any difficulties with mood or behavior.

Along with exercise, a **healthy diet** with less concentrated sugar and greater protein is important. Nourishing green vegetables and fruits that are rich in antioxidants are especially good. Such fruits as blackberries, raspberries, and particularly blueberries are smart choices because they are filled with flavonoid. A **flavonoid** is a type of antioxidant that acts as an anti-inflammatory that both aids in reducing fatigue and protects the brain against oxidative stress. Avocados, although quite pricey at the supermarket, are a sensible choice for brain health. They are full of folate, vitamins B, C, and E, and potassium, which increases blood flow to the brain and can lower one's heart rate. Protein, including fish, lean meats, nuts, and eggs, are alternatives to high-fat content meats such as ham, hotdogs, and spareribs. A diet high in fat will most likely exacerbate symptoms and increase flareups.

Lastly, patients should eat moderately. Overeating promotes lethargy and slows down brain function. Physicians should consider recommending that their patients eat by the clock. This can be easily taught by having them set a timer, watch alarm, or smartphone to alert them to when it is time to eat. Such a routine schedule helps the human body do better. At the same time, the doctor should monitor the patient's weight, which is easily done during routine visits. Studies have indicated that those with MTBI tend to gain weight.

Initiation & Planning

Initiation is the brain's ability to translate thoughts into an activity. An MTBI can weaken a person's capacity to initiate a task even though they may have gone to great lengths to plan and organize. To family and friends, this may look like a motivation problem, but, in fact, an inability to initiate is unrelated to energy level or ambition. Rather, the injury may have left the brain powerless to process specific detailed thought and turn it into activity. MTBI survivors face challenges to their reasoning and thought. Completing a single task involves a complex network of processes. If one is impaired, then receiving, comprehending, and acting appropriately causes a great deal of chaos when it comes to completing tasks, creating an executive functioning problem. To compensate, often MTBI patients will search out new methods in order to solve higher-level thinking problems.

Planning is the capacity to think ahead, whether that be for the next hour, day, month, or year. A patient cannot decide what to do or how to accomplish a task. Many who suffer from this problem have to rely on others to help make plans or simply stay within a repetitive routine.

Organization is the process of placing daily plans in order. For instance, it may involve taking your 4-year-old daughter to preschool, starting with fixing her breakfast and ending with dropping her off at the school. Initiation and organization are interlinked. Think of them as a husband and wife holding hands. One cannot be in a relationship without the other. Secondly, initiation and organization both require memory, problem solving, and sequencing. If you are unable to track and sequence the past, present, and future, it will appear as if somehow time has been lost. As a result, you will become overwhelmed emotionally and feel great anxiety that will aggravate the other MTBI symptoms.

An MTBI can impede your capability to carry out tasks that you have set out to do. Family and friends may perceive this as a motivational problem, which, of course, is far from the truth. In the MTBI world this is not an ambition problem but damage that affects translating the thought process and turning it into action. Recall our patient, Jenny. She was organized and quite successful at her work. She knew the tasks that needed to get done. Yet she did not reach the point of doing them. Sadly, such powerlessness to process information post injury is not readily apparent to the patient nor to the evaluating physician who is unaware of **ALL** the MTBI symptoms.

Many neuropsychologists and vocational rehabilitation counselors will evaluate your ability to process information by providing a neurological cognitive exam, which will reveal if an MTBI has affected speed, duration, and response time. Let's take a step back for a moment to consider what this is like. Imagine taking a cooking tray out of the oven without using a heat protective glove and not reacting to the heat that is burning your hand. Or picture a fire at a baseball stadium and not understanding why all the fans are clearing the ballpark and heading for the exits. It bears repeating again here: it is imperative for your general physician to refer both a neuropsychologist and vocational counselor to run a battery of tests and offer additional treatment that may be needed in order for you to get better. Most neuropsychologists and vocational counselors will be able to determine when you are able to return to your original life. It is important to keep in mind what Jenny was once told by her legal representative: "You must accept the fact that you might not get better. You probably will get better, but you might not now. The question for you, once you accept this, is to figure out who this "new person" you are is and what ride you can go on and enjoy *AS YOU ARE"* — Michael Richter, Attorney at Law and MTBI Survivor.

The Psychological Aspects of MTBI

The mental health aspects of MTBI are much more complicated to identify than are physical and emotional symptoms. We know where head or neck pain originates from. But if you are an MTBI patient having random acts of crying or angry outbursts, it is not so simple. The first phase in determining the origin is recognizing that what is happening to you is not an ordinary emotion. Then, overcome the embarrassment of discussing it with a treating provider. At that point, you have begun to overcome the hurdles you need to jump over prior to receiving treatment.

Depression

Depression is the single most common psychiatric disorder associated with MTBI and one of the most problematic for patients to recognize. An evaluating clinician who has identified their patient with depression should refer them for a psychologist's consultation or full treatment program that specializes in treating brain injuries. A specialist is the one who can best accomplish the difficult task of distinguishing between depression and other symptoms related to brain injury.

The complication lies in the fact that depression and the side effects of MTBI share numerous traits. Many times, depression creates a snowball effect that will aggravate MTBI symptoms (trouble concentrating, memory deficits, sleep disturbance, and fatigue). The list below contains the symptoms most associated with depression, symptoms that align with the side effects most related to an MTBI:

- Significant change in appetite
- Fatigue
- Apathy (lack of interest in everyday life)
- Self-loathing (the feeling of not being enough)
- Lack of sexual desire (decreased libido)
- Inability to feel pleasure (anhedonia)
- Lack of motivation
- Thoughts of suicide
- Feelings of helplessness
- Feelings of hopelessness

Even though there are many similarities between depression and MTBI, they are not one in the same. When the brain sustains trauma, more than likely neurochemical changes occur independently, linking them together. According to the *Quick Reference to the Diagnostic: Criteria from Diagnostic Statistical Manual of Mental Health Disorders* (American Psychiatric Association, 1994), to be classed as having a major depression disorder, a patient must have two or more of five symptoms for two weeks nearly every day for most of the day. One of these symptoms must be either a depressed mood or general loss of interest or pleasure.

You can, and should, take stock of what is going on with you. If you believe you are having one of the following symptoms, please take care of yourself by discussing it with your treating physician.

1. Depressed mood most of the day (feelings of sadness or emptiness)

2. Less than usual interest or pleasure in activities

3. Sleep disturbance (insomnia or hypersomnia)

4. Increased or decreased activity level

5. Change in appetite or significant weight gain (5 percent body weight in one month)

6. Fatigue or loss of energy

7. Excessive guilt or feelings of worthlessness

8. Poor concentration or indecisiveness

9. Recurrent thoughts of suicide or death

Depression Assessment for the MTBI Patient has been provided in **Appendix D** for the healthcare professional for use with their patients. This assessment tool can also be utilized as a portion of the clinical information submitted to the insurance company to obtain services for mental health. It has been modified from a geriatric depression scale (Sheikh et al. 1991; Yesavage et al. 1983; Brink et al. 1982).

Appendix D
Depression Assessment for the MTBI Patient

Answer the questions by checking **Yes** or **No** for each.

1. Do you feel dissatisfied with your life? Yes ◯   No ◯
2. Have you dropped many of your activities or interests? Yes ◯   No ◯
3. Do you feel that your life is empty? Yes ◯   No ◯
4. Do you often get bored? Yes ◯   No ◯
5. Do you feel your future is hopeless? Yes ◯   No ◯
6. Are you bothered by thoughts that you cannot get out of your head? Yes ◯   No ◯
7. Are you down and in poor spirits most of the time? Yes ◯   No ◯
8. Are you afraid something bad is going to happen to you? Yes ◯   No ◯
9. Do you feel sad most of the time? Yes ◯   No ◯
10. Do you often get restless or fidgety? Yes ◯   No ◯
11. Do you often feel helpless? Yes ◯   No ◯
12. Do you prefer to stay home rather than go out and do new things? Yes ◯   No ◯
13. Do you frequently worry about the future? Yes ◯   No ◯
14. Do you feel you have more problems with memory than most people? Yes ◯   No ◯
15. Do you think it is difficult and draining to be alive now? Yes ◯   No ◯
16. Do you often feel downhearted and blue? Yes ◯   No ◯
17. Do you feel worthless the way you are now? Yes ◯   No ◯
18. Do you worry a lot about the past? Yes ◯   No ◯
19. Do you feel life is dull and boring? Yes ◯   No ◯
20. Is it hard for you get a start on new projects? Yes ◯   No ◯
21. Are you lacking energy? Yes ◯   No ◯
22. Do you feel that your situation is hopeless? Yes ◯   No ◯
23. Do you feel that most people are better off than you are? Yes ◯   No ◯
24. Do you frequently get upset about things? Yes ◯   No ◯
25. Do you frequently feel like crying? Yes ◯   No ◯
26. Do you have trouble concentrating? Yes ◯   No ◯

27. Do you prefer to avoid social gatherings? Yes ○   No ○

28. Do you have trouble getting up in the mornings? Yes ○   No ○

29. Is it difficult for you to make decisions? Yes ○   No ○

30. Is your mind less clear than it used to be? Yes ○   No ○

Count the number of times that you answered *yes* to the above questions.

Total number of **Yes** answers: _____

If you answered **Yes** to **10** or more of the questions above, it is likely that you have depression. Please remember that this questionnaire does not take the place of a psychiatric evaluation. However, in conjunction with the information in the **Diagnostic and Statistical Manual of Mental Disorders, 4th Edition** or **DSM-IV** (the official source on definitions related to mental illness), it should give an idea of whether you are suffering from depression or not.

Imagine for a moment that you are someone suffering from depression as its own condition and are, at the same time, faced with symptoms from an MTBI. It can be very dangerous, because depression has a tendency to severely worsen the effects from a brain injury. So, it is a good idea for you to employ some coping strategies that can help in conjunction with the professional services of an astute psychologist.

Exercise: all physical activity has been known to help with decreasing irritability and a negative state of mind. It does not have to be strenuous—walking, hiking, gardening, or running—just meet the objective of being consistent. Outdoor activities are strongly recommended because they allow you to venture out of the house. Always remember to contact your physician prior to starting or resuming any physical activity, as the brain may still be tender from the injury.

Socialize: being around people and talking with others can be helpful when you are depressed. Your life may be struck with an MTBI, leaving you feeling isolated and alone. Because others do not understand the condition, you may not want to communicate with people. Do **NOT** let the MTBI be the reason why you cannot go see a movie with a relative, enjoy a cup of tea with your sister, or dial up an old friend you have not spoken to in years. It is healthy to open up to others about your MTBI and concerns about your depression. You never know. A family member or friend may have some good advice. Just keep in mind that the advice, whether you consider it or not and how therapeutic it may seem, does **NOT**, by any means, supplant the value of psychotherapy.

Counter negative thoughts: the biggest danger of MTBI depression is having so many negative thoughts that you feel hopeless and think that you will never get any better. To address this, your attending physician may refer you to a therapist who specializes in cognitive behavior therapy (CBT). While you wait to obtain insurance authorization for CBT and search for a contracted provider, both of which can be quite a process, your medical clinician may work with you on countering negative thoughts. It is a fairly simple process, really. First the patient is asked to monitor their negative thoughts by documenting them on paper. Secondly, the clinician assesses if there is any validity behind the negative thought. **Appendix E:** *How to Counter a Negative Thought* (based on Paterson, Randy, Your Depression Map, 2002, Publishers Group West) lays out the process.

Appendix E
How to Counter a Negative Thought

Take a moment to reflect on a negative thought you are having right now.

My negative thought is (write it here): _____

And the truth is: _____

If this thought is really true, these are steps I need to take in order to get better:

1. _____

2. _____

3. _____

4. _____

You will notice that the revised thought may **NOT** be as drastic as you originally believed. In fact, normally the reality is much less extreme than we had made it out to be.

It is far from easy to judge that you are in need of mental health services while struggling to accept the organic changes from a traumatic brain injury. Once you do, though, there are some ways to help yourself overcome MTBI depression:

1. See a therapist familiar with MTBI. Your doctor might suggest an on-line site or patient reviews through Yelp to help you decide on a therapist you would feel comfortable with. Ask during your initial intake process or first appointment.

2. After working awhile with your chosen therapist, if you do **NOT** feel comfortable, there is no reason to stay with them. Make sure that you can open up to them. If you cannot, the assistance that they can provide you with will be limited. Remember not to short-change yourself. That is to say, get the most you can out of every session, because your insurance will most likely pay for a limited number of therapy visits.

3. Be open and do not be afraid to ask questions. The more genuine and open you are, the greater benefit you will get out of therapy. Always remember that knowledge is power and that to become empowered you must express your fears and specific concerns. The more you discover about yourself, the better position you will be in as you progress.

"Keep hope alive" is the motto that can help you overcome symptoms for your MTBI. The steps you take towards getting better may not be at the pace that you or your loved ones are used to. Always be aware that you are trying to cope with some profoundly serious physical, mental, and psychological concerns. Hang onto hope. Even through those times when you find yourself questioning some of the deepest parts of yourself that can make you wonder why you are still alive. Always remember that you have a place in the world, and, with time, you will get better.

Anxiety

If depression is the "root," anxiety would be the "branches" and "vines" of an MTBI plant. Anxiety is a direct side effect of trauma to the brain. It is not abnormal to feel anxious when you try to focus and cannot remember. Furthermore, you may become sensitive to light or sound, which can lead to feeling stressed. When the body goes through physiological or organic changes, it can perceive that we are in danger, even if our life is not threatened. Because this danger is only a perception (we have no reason to fight or flee in most situations), we are left with anxiety.

The antonym (opposite word) for anxiety is relaxation. If you can learn how to "push the relaxation button" as an MTBI survivor, you may lessen your symptoms. Anxiety can interfere with attention, thus diminishing memory and cognition. As an illustration, our patient Jenny became anxious over missing work meetings and not remembering detailed information. This worsened her MTBI symptoms by increasing her head pain and fatigue. The good news for Jenny was that her psychologist, Dr. Framer, taught her relaxation techniques that made a big difference in her recovery.

The message of Jenny's success is that there is a way to cycle out of anxiety, through relaxation. Relaxation is more than lying on the couch and watching your favorite TV shows on Netflix. For the MTBI patient, relaxation is placing your mind at rest, thereby preventing the heightening of symptoms. Deep breathing exercises, muscle relaxation, and visualization exercises, all quite effective, can be easily learned by the patient and promotes a positive state of mind.

The healthcare professional can help you learn deep breathing exercises. They will begin with an explanation of deep breathing that will help your brain clam down, allowing a sense of calmness to be relayed throughout your entire body. Then they will help you find a quiet place in your home where you will not be distracted. Having a quiet place cannot be stressed enough for deep breathing to be most beneficial. Finally, once a calm place is determined, they will lead you through the six simple steps listed below:

1. Sit or stand with good posture or lie flat on the floor with your hand on your belly.

2. Inhale through your nose for four seconds and let your belly push your hand out.

3. Hold for four seconds.

4. Exhale through pursed lips for four seconds and feel the hand on your belly go in.

5. Hold for four seconds.

6. Repeat this cycle three to ten times daily.

Progressive muscle relaxation (PMR) is a second intervention for managing anxiety. It involves tensing and releasing the muscles. Through regular practice, muscle groups become unlocked from increased tension. The healthcare professional can easily teach PMR to the patient and, as "homework," can give the patient **Appendix F: *Progressive Muscle Relaxation Handout Sheet*** (www.biag.com.au/facts.htm, *Stress & Brain Injury*, October 2014. Brain Injury Association of Queensland, Australia).

Appendix F
Progressive Muscle Relaxation Handout Sheet

Focus upon 4 main muscle groups:

1. Hand, forearms, and biceps

2. Head, face, throat, and shoulders

3. Chest, stomach, and lower back

4. Thighs, buttocks, calves and feet

Tense muscles for 5–7 seconds and relax for 10–15 seconds.

Visualization is another approach. Unlike deep breathing exercises and progressive muscle relaxation, it does not have a physical component. When you daydream, this is visualization. The goal of this technique is to take your mind to a specific place in order to release tension.

Jenny's psychologist, Dr. Framer, taught her a semi-hypnosis approach called guided visualization. **Guided visualization** provides patients with a script of detailed meditation, possibly a scene walking on the beach or in a forest. With all the technology available on smart phones, it is quite easy to find audio scripts through Apple iPhone or Google Apps. *The Head Space: Meditation and Sleep* app is especially useful for MTBI patients, as it has reminders of specific days and times when to do a guided visualization exercise. The app also features a customized plan for those who are beginners to meditation versus the folks who have had experience with guided imagery exercises prior to injury. When coming out of a guided meditation exercise, it is strongly advised to come back gradually, on a count of 5, by slowly moving your arms and legs, saving the very last step to be slowly opening your eyes.

Identifying Anxiety for Patients with Post-Concussion Syndrome (PCS)

A healthcare professional will find the Beck's Anxiety Scale (BAI) invaluable when it comes to assisting with evaluating an MTBI patient's psychiatric symptoms. BAI has become the gold standard for the Veterans Affairs Administration Program (VA), evaluating an estimated 20,000 to 30,000 concussion-related accidents per year. The McGill University Traumatic Brain Injury Program observed acute levels of anxiety and depression in patients with MTBI despite the fact that neuropsychological scores remained within the normative zone. The patients themselves could see a cognitive decline while the neuropsychologist could not identify any problems correlated with the MTBI. However, the outcome from McGill University encourages administrators and clinicians to offer psychological support by a trained psychologist. As a result of receiving increased psychological support during the acute phase, the intensity of perceived post-concussive symptoms was drastically reduced, leading to a more favorable outcome (E. DeGuise, J. LeBlanc, S. Tinawi, J. Lamourex, and M. Feyz, *Acute Relationship between Cognitive and Psychological Symptoms of Patients with Mild Traumatic Brain Injury.* 2011. International Scholarly Research Notices, Vol. 2012, Article ID 147285).

One recommendation is to encourage health care administrators and providers to utilize the BAI scale, as the scores may assist in supporting a referral to a trained psychologist/counselor who would become actively involved with the patient's care early on versus waiting for post-concussion symptoms to fester. In **Appendix G: *Beck's Anxiety Scale (BAI)*** is made available for the healthcare clinician to further support the need for psychological services for the MTBI patient. (Source: Bluemtassoicates.com, Beck Anxiety Inventory(pdf), 2011/12. Blue Mountain Associates.)

Appendix G
Beck Anxiety Inventory (BAI)

Below is a list of common symptoms of anxiety. Please carefully read each item in the list. Indicate how much you have been bothered by that symptom during the past month, including today, by circling the number in the corresponding space in the column next to each symptom.

Bothered by symptom	Not at all	Mildly; it didn't bother me much	Moderately; it wasn't pleasant at times	Severely; it bothered me a lot
Numbness or tingling	0	1	2	3
Feeling hot	0	1	2	3
Wobbliness in legs	0	1	2	3
Unable to relax	0	1	2	3
Fear of worst happening	0	1	2	3
Heart pounding/racing	0	1	2	3
Unsteady	0	1	2	3
Terrified	0	1	2	3
Nervous	0	1	2	3
Feeling of choking	0	1	2	3
Hands trembling	0	1	2	3
Shaky/unsteady	0	1	2	3
Fear of losing control	0	1	2	3
Difficulty in breathing	0	1	2	3
Fear of dying	0	1	2	3
Scared	0	1	2	3
Indigestion	0	1	2	3
Faint/lightheaded	0	1	2	3
Face flushed	0	1	2	3
Hot/cold sweats	0	1	2	3
Column Sum				

Scoring: Sum each column. Then sum the column totals to achieve a grand score.

Write the **grand score** here: _____

Interpretation

A grand score between **0–21** indicates very low anxiety, usually a good thing. Still, it is possible that either you might be unrealistic in your assessment, which would be denial, or that you have learned to mask the symptoms associated with anxiety. Some anxiety can be expected. Too little anxiety could indicate that you are detached from yourself, others, or your environment.

A grand score between **22–35** indicates moderate anxiety. Your body is trying to tell you something. Look for patterns as to when and why you experience the symptoms described above. For instance, if it occurs prior to public speaking and your job requires a lot of presentations, you will want to find ways to calm yourself before speaking or let others do some of the presentations. You may have some conflict issues that need to be resolved. Clearly, it is not panic time, but you do want to find ways to manage the stress you feel.

A grand score that exceeds **36** is a potential cause for concern. Again, look for patterns or times when you tend to feel the symptoms you have circled as severe. Persistent and high anxiety is not a sign of personal weakness or failure. It is, though, something that needs to be proactively treated or there could be a significant negative impact to you mentally and physically. You may want to consult a counselor if the feelings persist.

Sports-Related Concussions

Although motor vehicle accidents and falls are responsible for the preponderance of concussions or mild traumatic brain injuries per year, the U.S. Centers for Disease Control and Prevention (CDC) estimates that 1.6 million sports-related concussions occur per year throughout the United States. The most startling statistic of all is that an estimated 283,000 children per year seek care in a U.S. emergency room for sports or recreational-related activities. Some 45% of those children seeking care for MTBI have sustained injuries from contact sports. Football, bicycling, and playground activities accounted for the highest number of emergency department visits. Certainly, efforts to improve safety for specific sports and recreation-related activities are crucial to reducing the risk for childhood MTBI (Kelly Sarmiento, Karen Thomas, Jill Daugherty, et al. *Emergency Department Visits for Sport and Recreation-Related Traumatic Brain Injuries Among Children–United States. 2010–2016.* MMWR Morb Mortal Wkly. Rep. March 2019/68 [10]).

Technology is advancing, like the modern football helmet, which does protect the exterior of the skull. Yet, inside, with acceleration or deceleration of the cranium, the brain bangs and rattles, and muscle fiber tissues are stretched, torn, and bruised. This trauma **cannot** be detected by an MRI or CT scan. As Dr. Ann McKee of Boston University School of Medicine has established, multiple head trauma produces a buildup of tau protein that becomes toxic in neurodegenerative diseases (e.g., Alzheimer's, Dementia, Huntington's, Parkinson's, and Spinocerebellar ataxia). When the brain experiences repeated blows to the head (chronic traumatic encephalopathy, or CTE), profound quantities of tau protein molecules clump and slowly start to accumulate throughout the entire brain, first in the brain's cortex, then around blood vessels, and, finally, very deep in the cortical sulci. The blending of tau will collect in the hippocampus (involved in learning and memory) and amygdala (involved with decision-making and emotions). Lastly, tau protein becomes very dense, covering the brain's cortex and other regions, including the spinal cord. Thus, the reason that so many college and NFL coaches have spoken up against youth under the age of 15 participating in football. In fact, the University of Michigan's football head coach, Jim Harbaugh, recommends that youth under the age of 15 play soccer instead, a sport very similar to football.

Contact in certain sports is unavoidable, and injuries should be watched for. A large variety of tests are in use that can determine if damage has happened. Because those tests can be confusing and seem complicated to people unfamiliar with them, some of the ones you may encounter are explained below.

Some tests can be administered on the sidelines. The most familiar concussion sideline test for athletes is the SCAT (Sport Concussion Assessment Tool)-3. Its objective is to quickly assess whether a player can return to the game or needs further evaluation. It includes a symptom checklist, and it tests for memory and cognitive changes. A sample portion of the SCAT-3 test is presented in **Appendix H: *SCAT-3 Symptom Evaluation.***

Despite having a SCAT-3 or Child SCAT-3 (available for those 13 years and younger), neuro-ophthalmological testing appears to be lacking in sideline assessments. Many sideline tests such as the SCAT-3 ask questions and observe the player's thinking, feeling, and walking. But athletes will tell the sideline healthcare professional, sports medicine specialist, or parent volunteer that they are "okay" so they will be allowed to return to the game.

The reality is that many symptoms cannot be noticed until the person tries to get back into a regular routine. A 12-year-old boy who sustained a possible concussion in the summertime may not recognize that he has a problem until he goes back to school in the fall, when school-work requires him to use different parts of his brain. Basically, the boy can pass the SCAT-3 remarkably, but not know there is a problem until his visual system has to deal with academics.

One sideline test that has demonstrated success is the King-Devick (K-D) test (see **Appendix I:** **_King-Devick Test_**). It was originally designed by a team of optometrists to evaluate children for dyslexia by gauging the amount of time it takes to read numbers on three cards. What is exciting about having the K-D test on the sidelines is that it integrates testing of attention, saccades (a rapid movement of the eyes that cannot respond to the change of position), and visual interpretation. And it can easily be administered on the sidelines by a parent or volunteer. Other batteries of tests do not capture the neurological systems, especially not fully evaluating the brainstem and cerebral cortex function.

Technically, every athlete who is diagnosed with a concussion should be prohibited from re-entering the game, but, as we all know, that does not always happen, especially with competitive leagues starting at such an early age and continuing all the way through college. A combination of the SCAT 3 in conjunction with the K-D test adds another layer of testing to proactively identify concussion-like symptoms. Sideline testing is very important, because delaying treatment of any brain injury will slow down the recovery process and place the patient at greater risk for post-concussion syndrome (PCS).

Appendix H

SCAT (Sport Concussion Assessment Tool) - 3 Symptom Evaluation

	None		Mild		Moderate		Severe
Headache	0	1	2	3	4	5	6
"Pressure in head"	0	1	2	3	4	5	6
Neck pain	0	1	2	3	4	5	6
Nausea or vomiting	0	1	2	3	4	5	6
Dizziness	0	1	2	3	4	5	6
Blurred vision	0	1	2	3	4	5	6
Balance problems	0	1	2	3	4	5	6
Sensitivity to light	0	1	2	3	4	5	6
Sensitivity to noise	0	1	2	3	4	5	6
Feel slowed down	0	1	2	3	4	5	6
Feel "in a fog"	0	1	2	3	4	5	6
"Don't feel right"	0	1	2	3	4	5	6
Cannot concentrate	0	1	2	3	4	5	6
Poor recall/low energy	0	1	2	3	4	5	6
Confusion	0	1	2	3	4	5	6
Drowsiness	0	1	2	3	4	5	6
Can't fall asleep	0	1	2	3	4	5	6
More emotional	0	1	2	3	4	5	6
Irritability	0	1	2	3	4	5	6
Sadness	0	1	2	3	4	5	6
Nervous/anxious	0	1	2	3	4	5	6

Total number of symptoms (max. 21): _____

Symptoms severity score (max. 126): _____

Do the symptoms get worse with physical activity? Yes ◌ No ◌

Do the symptoms get worse with mental activity? Yes ◌ No ◌

Self-rated and clinician-monitored ◌   Self-rated ◌

Self-rated with parent input ◌   Clinician interview ◌

Note: This is a sample portion of the exam and should **not** be used as a stand-alone method for diagnosing a concussion.

Source: Adapted from British Journal of Sports Medicine

Appendix I
King-Devick (K-D) Test

1. Have the athlete read numbers left to right on each card as quickly as possible without making any errors.

2. Use a stopwatch when the subject reads the first number and stop when the last number is read.

3. Record time in seconds using the stopwatch. The K-D time is based on the cumulative amount of time it takes to complete all three test cards.

4. The total score is based on the sum of each of the three test cards.

5. Record the number of errors reading the test cards.

6. Record misspeaks on numbers as errors if the subject does not immediately correct the mistake before continuing to the next number.

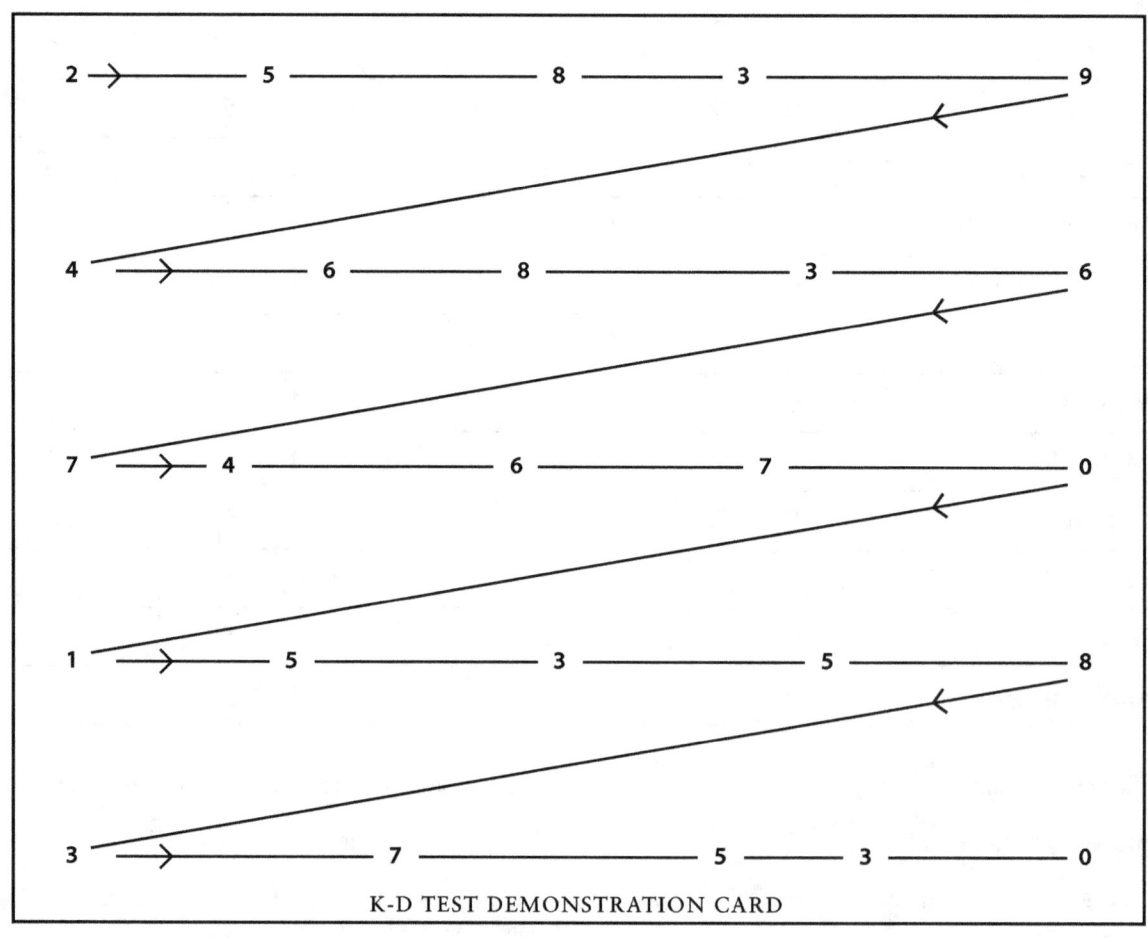

K-D TEST DEMONSTRATION CARD

2 ——————— 5 ——————— 8 ——— 0 ——————— 7

3 ——— 7 ——————— 9 ——————————— 4 ——————— 6

5 ——————— 3 ——————————— 1 ——————— 6 ——————— 4

7 ——————————— 9 ——————— 7 ——————— 3 ——————— 5

1 ——————— 5 ——————————— 4 ——————————— 9 ——————— 2

6 ——————————— 5 ——————— 5 ——————————— 7 ——— 3

3 ——— 1 ——————————— 8 ——————————— 6 ——————— 4

5 ——————————————— 3 ——————————— 7 ——— 5 ——————— 2

K-D TEST I

---

3   7   5   9   0

2   5   7   4   6

1   4   7   6   3

7   9   3   9   0

4   5   2   1   7

5   3   7   4   8

7   4   6   5   2

9   0   2   3   6

K-D TEST II

49

```
5          4          1               8               0
4          6                    3          5          9
7          5                      4    2          7
3     2          6               9          4
1          4          5          1          3
9               3     4               8          5
5     1               6               3     1
4          3          5     2          7
```

K-D TEST III

Neurological Testing for MTBI

Many doctors will order an **MRI (magnetic resonance imaging)** or **CT (computed tomography) scan.** Unfortunately, neither of these detects a concussion to the brain, although they can rule out a tumor, brain bleed, or aneurysm. These types of scans are a very useful resource to detect physical or structural changes to the brain, but they fall short in revealing damaged neurons, blood vessels, and overall energy that is required to keep the brain functioning. Interestingly enough, many different types of testing are available that may reveal what part of the brain is damaged. A **SPECT (single-photon emission computed tomography) scan** will display an actual 3-D picture of the brain. A SPECT scan shows what part of the brain is active or less active by injecting a small amount of radioactive substance that is traced through the brain. SPECT scans can be extremely helpful to physicians by determining what parts of the brain are affected by dementia, epilepsy, seizures, clogged blood vessels, and head injuries. Consequently, the SPECT scan can give physicians essential information to share with their patients, and, most importantly, confirm if brain dysfunction has occurred after a concussion.

An **fMRI (functional magnetic resonance imaging) scan**, a fourth option, works through a combination of radio waves and magnets. Radio waves are able to form a 3D image of the brain's tissues and reveal any physical damage sustained by observing blood flow. This means that an fMRI can demonstrate detailed images of blood flow in internal organs, observe how the brain is managing oxygen supply, and determine whether the right regions respond when given a certain task. For example, a post-concussion syndrome (PCS) scan may show telltale signs of hyperactivity and hypoactivity in the affected regions of the brain. This information will allow the doctor to pinpoint a treatment plan, as the brain and its dysfunction are immediately visible. On the other hand, many considerations come into play when calculating the accuracy of a scan. First and foremost, case studies have focused primarily on patients who are within the mean of 20 to 30 years old; therefore, the data cannot adequately address age variations in functional brain changes after an injury. Equally important, most research has touched solely on the subacute post-injury period (1 to 2 months post-injury). The brain's chemistry post-injury shifts over time, altering damaged regions and restricting blood flow, so an fMRI may not present an accurate picture of the patient's current condition (Brenna McDonald, Andrew Saykin, and Thomas McAllister. *Functional MRI of mild traumatic brain injury (MTBI): progress and perspectives from the first decade of studies.* Brain Imaging and Behavior, Volume 6, 193–207 (2012) https://doi.org/10.1007/s11682-012-9173-4).

The most thorough scan a patient with a MTBI can receive is an **fNCI (functional neurovascular coupling imaging) scan.** This is an advanced form of a fMRI that has been standardized for clinical application. The scan entails imaging and testing from six different cognitive tests performed inside an MRI machine. An fNCI takes over 7000 images in a 40-minute window, giving near real-time images that measure the connection between the brain and blood in the brain. By processing these images, it tells the doctor the severity of an injury in each region of the brain. Neurovascular coupling (NVC) is the connection between neurons (brain cells) and blood vessels. Neurons need blood vessels to supply them with energy in order to do their job. When an injury or neurological disorder occurs, the connection between blood vessels and neurons is strained. As a result, the brain does not provide enough energy to function. If the brain does not receive the correct amount of energy, it triggers such symptoms as fatigue, headaches, attention difficulties, memory issues, sleep problems, and emotional distress. Allowing these symptoms to fester for greater than six weeks with either no treatment or the wrong type of treatment puts the patient at a very high risk for post-concussion syndrome (PCS). The benefit of a neurovascular scan is that it will show where the lack of blood flow is in the brain and give the patient a chance for proactive treatment that may consist of physical, cognitive, and motor exercises. Providing a patient with a weekly rehabilitation program reduces concussion symptoms by restoring healthy NVC, hence producing a positive outcome.

Healthcare Coverage & Disability Insurance

One of the biggest challenges of any injury is being cognizant of what aspects of health care your insurance policy covers—what you can get them to authorize. Right away, you need to determine what type of policy will be responsible for the injury. Insurance policies (types of plans) vary, such as an indemnity plan (auto insurance or Workers' Compensation) or strictly a healthcare plan. Although both may cover an injury, depending on the circumstances, auto insurance usually has a cap of a certain dollar amount, like $20,000 for personal injury, and the amount may differ, based on if you are at fault. Then there is second party insurance, which changes the picture entirely. Auto insurance carriers are delegated to make a referral to what is called **utilization review (U/R)**. U/R is done by independent companies that are comprised of physicians and case managers who review the medical records (clinical information) to determine whether certain services (physical therapy, chiropractic care, medications, etc.) can be authorized because they meet the definition of medical necessity. You will have a right to appeal any decision made by U/R, and that is discussed later. For now, clearly understand that U/R is in place to contain costs for the insurance company; they are **NOT** your advocate.

In the world of auto insurance, an adjustor can easily override a U/R decision, unlike its "300-pound sister," better known as Workers' Compensation. An employer does not himself pay for an injured worker but does have Workers' Compensation insurance coverage. The bad news is that the Workers' Compensation system is a nightmare, being the most underregulated in the healthcare industry. Healthcare providers, such as those in the fields of occupational medicine and urgent care, receive reimbursement from that agency for medically managing the injured worker. Truth be told, unscrupulous doctors in occupational medicine are, for lack of a better word, "hacks" for the insurance company. This means that they will evaluate the patient and report using certain medical terms that will favor the criteria of the Workers' Compensation carrier over the patient. Such terms as "no longer making progress," "therapeutic goals have been reached," "okay to transition to the next level of care," "patient will no longer benefit from," and "services are not medically necessary" are catch phrases that make it difficult for even an appeal by an independent reviewer to go in the patient's favor.

It's important to remember that patients have the right to select their own doctor to medically manage their condition. Employers will encourage the injured worker to be treated at their contracted occupational medicine clinic, but this is **NOT** a good idea, especially for those who have sustained a brain injury. As an injured worker, you have a right to seek a medical evaluation from a physician of your choice. Another of your rights is to appeal the denial of any medications or services that have been denied. **Warning:** the risk with an appeal is that if the decision is not overturned in your favor, the requested medications or services cannot be submitted again for an entire year from the date of denial. If at any time you are uncertain about your rights or do not know where to begin to find a treating physician to take care of you, **The Brain Injury Association of America** (www.biusa.org) can help you navigate through the process.

After a work-related injury, the time and procedures for filing a claim differ from state-to-state. Under Workers' Compensation law, you are entitled to medications that are related to the injury, plus treatment such as physical, occupational, and speech therapy, as well as a percentage of your pre-injury earnings. If the insurance carrier's physician does not submit a report substantiating your injury, you may not be covered but instead forced back to work prematurely. Unsurprisingly, this will spiral your condition and place you at greater risk for post-concussion syndrome (PCS). At this point, you might want to seek legal counsel or locate a qualified practitioner who understands MTBI (your local **Brain Injury Association** can help). Overall, do keep in mind during the process that, once approved, payments from Workers' Compensation take time and do not happen right away.

The lucky ones have checked the box for disability insurance. **Disability coverage** will pay a percentage of your current wages while you are disabled. Many companies offer this for their employees, so, before you suffer an injury, it is best to check with your employer to confirm if you have coverage or not. Your employer will provide you with an application and instructions needed to file a claim.

Several government programs are available that may provide benefits to people with MTBI. Programs that you may find applicable are **Social Security Disability Insurance (SSDI), Supplemental Security Income (SSI),** and the **Veterans Affairs Administration Program (VA).** Know that medical assistance is a combination of state and federal benefits; there could be restrictions on coverage of types of treatment, medication, and equipment.

SSDI would be the first place I would recommend to apply. It is applicable for those who were employed for a required period of time. Legal advocates can help you file an application but will take a percentage of the maximum payment allowed by law from the initial settlement. They offer aid with completing the application, and they advocate for you when you require legal assistance to appeal an SSDI denial.

Conversely, if you have never been employed or have extraordinarily little income, SSI is a possibility. Your local government offices can assist in completing the application for both SSI and SSDI. Do **NOT** expect payment from either of these programs to occur immediately. In many cases, the application process itself can take up to three years. Once accepted, though, benefits are retroactive, which means that if you do receive SSDI or SSI, you will be reimbursed from the day of injury.

In most states, VA hospitals have knowledgeable physicians on staff that are quite savvy in treating brain injuries. If you served in the military and have become disabled, you may be eligible for wage or medical assistance. To apply for benefits, contact the nearest Veterans Administration office.

As you can see, the journey for obtaining healthcare and financial coverage can be very intimidating. Do **NOT** let that stop you. The insurance provider may like you give up so they do not have to pay for your care. Do not be discouraged; get help from others, starting with your local **Brain Injury Association**. Your spouse or family members can help out with tasks like making different folders and filing information that has been sent to you by each provider. Help yourself, as well. Document the date, time, and what has been said during each and every communication with an insurance plan or social security representative. Stand up for your right to request medical records from your doctors or treating specialist, such as a psychologist or physical therapist. You will need this information to make sure that the appropriate medical records get to the individuals who are making the decisions, or you could be denied for what is called "lack of clinical," meaning that your health plan or government agency did not receive all the medical records needed in order to approve the benefit. As a Workers' Compensation patient, you may be subject to independent medical evaluations (IME) or vocational rehabilitation consultations, possibly by providers being paid by the insurance company, so do not expect a favorable evaluation. And have legal representation that can advocate for your medical and financial wellbeing. An attorney who specializes in working with the brain injured can secure not only medical benefits but a financial settlement for your loss, especially if you are not able to return to work.

A Blueprint for Family & Friends

An MTBI impacts everyone who relates to the patient. Family and friends who are involved with their loved one on a regular basis can affect the recovery process either positively or negatively, based on how they respond to the brain injured individual. The key thought to remember is patience, patience, patience.

As family or friend, the person they once knew may not exist any longer. They may observe that the person they have known for all these years is exhibiting strange behavior that makes no sense at all. Someone who was once sharp and articulate with an excellent memory now asks to repeat the same thing over again three to five times. This new person might be more likable than before, or they may not be very likeable at all. Family and friends see the person as a stranger, feel that they have lost a loved one, and go through the stages of grief. Through it all, they should try to imagine how that loved one is feeling and practice patience, patience, patience.

Obviously, living with a person overcoming an MTBI is not easy. You can help yourself and your loved one by attending physician appointments and asking plenty of questions regarding certain behavioral and other problems that you may have encountered. Educate yourself about the deficits, tests, and exercises described in this playbook. Recognize that an MTBI passes through different phases of recovery. Learn about each phase and devise an approach for coping with it. Always address a person who has an MTBI by name, especially before asking to do something that you would like them to remember. Understand that there is nothing wrong with talking openly to others regarding the "old" person and frustration with this "new" person that you have been gifted with.

Get to know the new person. Accept your feelings of frustration and anger toward them as normal and find others through support groups, either in person or on social media. Reach out to your friend or family member by taking walks through the neighborhood, or go grab a cup of coffee at a quiet place. Discover what community services are available that can aid people with MTBI in the home or workplace, then discuss them with your loved one. Try to focus on the positive, such as the strengths and talents that your loved one still possesses. Sometimes you will find yourself in disagreement and emotional distress. Do not despair but consider personal, couple, or family counseling. Once again, a great place to start if you are feeling the pressure of being solely in charge of your loved one's recovery is to call or email your state **Brain Injury Association** or the national office of the **Brain Injury Association of America** for advice and referrals.

Another excellent tool to further understand an MTBI is through the *Mild Traumatic Brain Injury: Wellness Zones* (see **Appendix J**). This is a model that was created for those who either do not understand brain injuries or struggle with acceptance, making it useful for patients, their families, and their friends. An invisible injury is difficult for everyone—the injured person, friends, family, and even for many doctors. The MTBI: Wellness Zones brings to light somewhat of a physicality of the symptoms that cannot be seen but experienced by an MTBI survivor on a regular basis.

Appendix J
Mild Traumatic Brain Injury: Wellness Zones

Green Zone
→ High Functioning.

→ Mild Symptoms – feels like you are able to walk through a grass field with ease.

→ Able to work and do house chores to the best of your capability.

→ Attend family and social activities.

Having a good day consists of the following:

★ Utilize the pace method.

★ Avoid loud and enclosed spaces that can make you tire easily.

★ Setting boundaries with family and friends in advance, prior to a social function.

★ Remember to take at least a 30 minute nap during the day, especially if you plan to go to an activity that is in the late afternoon or evening.

★ Taking as many breaks and finding a quiet place as needed.

★ Pack a survival bag: water, snacks, heat and ice packs, neck pillow, and a ball or sun hat.

★ Do **NOT** forget your adaptive devices: hearing aid and filters, photophobia eyeglasses.

★ Take medications and use your TENS (transcutaneous electrical nerve stimulation) Unit as prescribed by your physician.

★ At least 30 – 45 minutes of exercise or as recommended by your doctor or physical therapist.

Yellow Zone
✳ Moderately intense symptoms.

✳ Taking more time than usual to track and follow social interaction.

✳ Increasing hypersensitivity to light and sound.

✳ Ear ringing (tinnitus) flares up much more than usual.

✳ You are at the point where the fake smile becomes a mask hiding how you are really feeling inside.

✳ Your brain tells you that it is time to sleep.

✳ Neck and shoulder muscles begin to tighten up more than usual.

✳ Pain levels on the **numeric rating scale (NRS)** are escalating.

✳ Finding that you are taking much more "as needed" pain medication.

Red Zone

- ✖ Severe intense symptoms.
- ✖ You want a quiet environment.
- ✖ Feeling as if you would like to hide in a rabbit hole and need sleep to recharge.
- ✖ Cannot find a balance between pain and fatigue.
- ✖ Too exhausted to follow 1:1 social interaction.
- ✖ Double vision becomes much more apparent.
- ✖ Movement and range of motion of neck and shoulders is much more restricted than usual.
- ✖ Pain is intensified to the point of preventing you from work, household chores, and social activities.
- ✖ Sudden alteration of mood and behavior – much more angry or irritable than usual.

I understand that fighting an invisible illness is life-threatening.

Signature: ____

Date: ____________

Conclusion

The recovery from a mild traumatic brain injury will not happen on the patient's or the medical professional's terms. The brain is an organ that will heal at its own pace. Immediately treating psychological needs will undoubtedly help lessen many symptoms being experienced by MTBI survivors. Nonetheless, the dilemma for the patient is finding a savvy physician who specializes in treating mild traumatic brain injuries and who has a clear understanding of how cerebral blood flow functions. When healthcare professionals are not up-to-date on the current literature, prompt medical attention is not given. Such a delay can create psychosocial factors that range from homelessness, to alcohol and drug addiction, to loss of spouse and employment.

As for treating providers, they need to take measures to collaborate and consult with each other, especially when establishing a treatment plan. They must recognize that the MTBI patient's life may spiral from every psychosocial aspect, whether that is loss of independence, alienation from spouse through separation or divorce, financial hardship from loss work, or inadequate housing. The lack of an established treatment plan can bring about any of these. Moreover, many of these psychosocial factors can be eliminated or at least mitigated if the healthcare provider is thoroughly educated in the treatment of MTBI.

We can hope that new technological advances for early treatment, such as the SPECT scan and off-counter approaches with prescribed medications, will continue to produce the necessary therapeutic steps towards early healing and recovery for future traumatic brain injury survivors. Meanwhile, the information contained in this playbook can empower patients, caregivers, and physicians to improve the MTBI's health and wellbeing.

A Personal Note

Approximately five years ago I sustained a mild traumatic brain injury (MTBI) that ultimately led me down the dark pathway of post-concussion syndrome (PCS). I am currently continuing to receive treatment from my physicians, who specialize in the field of mild and traumatic brain injuries. It had taken me over a year post-injury to find them, and I am forever grateful. My life has changed. Even though I no longer can do everything I did before my injury, I have much more appreciation for what I can do right now.

—Sean Mullins

Resources

Allen, PhD, Mark. *fMRI vs. SPECT Scan for the Brain: Know Your Options*. 2020. Provo, UT. https://www.cognitivefxusa.com

Davies, NCTMB, Clair and Amber Davies, CMTPT, LMT. *The Trigger Point Therapy Workbook Third Eddition*. 2013. New Harbinger Publications, Oakland, CA.

DeGuise, E., J. LeBlanc, S. Tinawi, J. Lamourex, and M. Feyz, *Acute Relationship between Cognitive and Psychological Symptoms of Patients with Mild Traumatic Brain Injury*. 2011. International Scholarly Research Notices, Vol. 2012, Article ID 147285

Keatley, PhD, CCC, Mary Ann and Laura Whittemore. *Understanding Mild Traumatic Brain Injury (MTBI)*. 2016. Brain Injury Hope Foundation, Boulder, CO.

Mason, PsyD, Douglas J. *The Mild Traumatic Injury Workbook*. 2002. New Harbinger Publications, Oakland, CA.

McDonald, Brenna, Andrew Saykin, and Thomas McAllister. *Functional MRI of mild traumatic brain injury (MTBI): progress and perspectives from the first decade of studies*. 2012. Brain Imaging and Behavior, Volume 6, 193–207. https://doi.org/10.1007/s11682-012-9173-4

Marshall, Cameron, Howard Vernon, John Leddy, and Bradley Baldwin. *The Role of the Cervical Spine in Post-Concussion Syndrome*. June 2015. The Physician and Sportsmedicine; 1–11.

Mayo Clinic Staff. *Convergence Insufficiency*. 2019. Mayo Foundation for Medical Education and Research (MFMER), Rochester, MN.

Oh, Joo Youn, Gavin W. Roddy, Hosoon Choi, Ryang Hwa Lee, Joni H. Ylöstalo, Robert H. Rosa Jr., and Darwin J. Prockop. *Anti-Inflammatory Protein TSG-6 Reduces Inflammatory Damage to the Cornea Following Chemical and Mechanical Injury*. 2010. PNAS September 28, 2010 107 (39) 16875-16880; 1012451107.

Sarmiento, Kelly, Karen Thomas, Jill Daughtery, et al. *Emergency Department Visits for Sport and Recreation-Related Traumatic Brain Injuries Among Children–United States*. 2010–2016. MMWR Morb Mortal Wkly Rep 2019; 68237-242. https://dx.doi.org/10.15585/mmwr.mm6810a2

Stoler, EdD, Diane Roberts, and Barbara Albers Hill. *Coping with Concussion and Mild Traumatic Brain Injury*. 1998. Penguin Group (USA), New York, NY. https://www.penguin.com

Stoler, EdD, Diane Roberts, and Barbara Albers Hill. *Coping with Mild Traumatic Brain Injury*. 2018. The Staywell Company, Yardley, PA.

Stuart, Ann. *Concussion Care*. December 2016. EyeNet Magazine, San Francisco, CA.

Vestibular Disorders Association. *How Do I Know if I Have a Vestibular Disorder?* 2016. Vestibular Disorders Association (VEDA), Portland, OR.

Index